The Visual Aural Digit Span Test

The Visual Aural Digit Span Test

Elizabeth Munsterberg Koppitz, Ph.D.
Board of Cooperative Educational Services
Yorktown Heights, New York.

(G&S)

GRUNE & STRATTON, INC.
Harcourt Brace Jovanovich, Publishers
Orlando   New York   San Diego   Boston   London
San Francisco   Tokyo   Sydney   Toronto

Library of Congress Cataloging in Publication Data

Koppitz, Elizabeth Munsterberg.
   The visual aural digit span test.

   Bibliography: p.
   Includes index.
   1. Learning disabilities.   2.   Ability—Testing.
I.   Title.
LC4704.K66   370.15′2   77-24889
ISBN 0-8089-1032-9

Grune & Stratton, Inc.
Orlando, FL 32887

Distributed in the United Kingdom by
Grune & Stratton, Ltd.
24/28 Oval Road, London NW 1

Library of Congress Catalog Number 77-24889
International Standard Book Number 0-8089-1032-9
Printed in the United States of America
          88   89   10 9 8 7 6

To my friends and colleagues on Tuder's team:
Lenny, April, Bill, Bob, Carol,
Helen, Jean, Jerry, John,
Madeline, Marie, Nancy,
Ruth, Sandra, Tom,
and all the
others

Table of Contents

List of Tables and Figures

FIGURES

Preface

For more than 15 years I have worked as a school psychologist with learning disabled youngsters. During this time I have become increasingly aware of the close relationship between children's reading, spelling and arithmetic achievement and their functioning in intersensory integration and recall. I have encountered many pupils with good visual and auditory perception who had difficulty with reading and spelling because of problems with symbol-sound association and with the sequencing of symbols and sounds. Other children who failed to show good progress in their school work appeared to be able to learn new information but they had difficulty remembering what they learned.

A meaningful psychologocial evaluation of school children has to include, therefore, measures of intersensory integration, sequencing, and recall. Such measures are, of course, included in the Wechsler and Stanford-Binet Scales, but it is not always feasible to give youngsters a full scale intelligence test when screening school beginners, or when diagnosing specific learning difficulties, or when assessing pupils' rates of progress. There is a need for a brief, easy to administer, reliable, standardized test of intersensory integration and memory for school children. Since I was unable to find such a test I decided to develop a test of my own. The Visual Aural Digit Span Test or VADS Test is the outcome of this effort.

I have used the VADS Test extensively in my work with elementary and middle school pupils and have found it to be a very useful and practical diagnostic instrument. A number of other psychologists and diagnosticians, who made use of the Experimental Edition of the VADS Test, have also expressed enthusiasm for the test and have urged me to publish my findings.

The VADS Test is easy to administer. It requires a minimum of equipment and takes only a few minutes to complete, yet it yields a considerable amount of information. The eleven different VADS Test measures include scores for both auditory and visual processing and recall, and for intrasensory integration and intersensory integration. The VADS Test scores of children, age 5½ to 12, can be compared with the test scores of other pupils of the same age or grade level, and the VADS Test score pattern can be analyzed for specific diagnostic clues or indicators. In addition, the VADS Test records can be evaluated for the organization and quality of the written digit sequences.

The VADS Test is presented here in the hope that it will help clinical and school psychologists, and diagnosticians working with children, to better understand youngsters' learning problems. It is also hoped that this book will stimulate further research with the VADS Test. Although a considerable amount of research data has accumulated, there are, so far, only a few published studies on the VADS Test. A great deal more research is needed to explore and to realize the full potential of this new and promising test.

This book was made possible because of the cooperation and support I received from many people. I am grateful to them all. Above all I want to thank my husband Werner who contributed to the research and who was always available for counsel; moreover, he endured with fortitude the stress of living with an author. I am also greatly indepted to the principals and teachers who permitted me to give the VADS Test to the youngsters in their classes in order to collect data for the normative sample, and to my friends and colleagues who shared with me their VADS Test data and research findings. Among these I would like to mention especially; Kay Butler, Margaret Carr, Serena Deutsch, Fred Fanning, Bianca Hirsch, Ann Hurd, Alma Jones, Michele Millavec, William Morea, James Nutt, Barbara Rubin, Doris Schwartz, Wayne Starch, Billy Watson, and Belle Ruth Witkin. I deeply appreciate the assistance I received from Barbara Ayers and Helen Maloney of the BOCES library who located and obtained for me many articles and reprints. My thanks also goes to Sally Roach who helped with the preparation of the manuscript. And finally I am grateful to the boys and girls who participated in the studies and who taught me so much.

Mt. Kisco, N.Y.
February, 1977
                                                        Elizabeth M. Koppitz

The Visual Aural Digit Span Test

Chapter 1

Introduction

Children's success or failure in school results from a combination and interaction of many different factors within the pupils themselves, and in their homes and schools. Efforts to attribute learning difficulties of schoolchildren to one specific problem, such as poor visual perception, mixed dominance, emotional maladjustment, distractibility, social deprivation, hyperactivity, speech problems, incoordination, lack of motivation, or a particular teaching method, have proven unsuccessful. Although all of these factors undoubtedly influence achievement, none of them, by itself, can account for a child's severe reading problems or failure in arithmetic.

It is now generally accepted that learning disabilities have no single cause, but rather are produced by a variety of problems that occur simultaneously. My own experience and research have convinced me that children's age, sex, visual-motor perception, mental ability, language skills, emotional adjustment, attitudes and values, motivation, developmental and medical histories, social background, and the educational program to which they have been exposed all contribute to their academic progress and functioning in school. In addition, I have become increasingly aware of the enormous importance of intersensory integration and recall for school achievement.

In the five year follow-up study of children with learning disabilities (Koppitz, 1971) I found that the pupils who showed the best progress and returned to regular classes, after a period in special classes, not only had good mental ability but also showed good intersensory integration and were able to retain what they learned. On the other hand, the four groups of learning-disabled youngsters who required long-term special education had serious problems in the areas of integration and recall.

The first group of these long-term special education pupils were above all slow. But in addition to poor reasoning ability, they also had serious problems with retaining from one day to the next what they learned. Baumeister et al. (1963) have shown that poor memory is an important factor in the limited achievement of slow youngsters.

The second group of educationally handicapped pupils also had difficulty with abstract reasoning and integration, but their visual memory for words was good. They belonged to that group of children that Silberberg and Silberberg (1967) called "hyperlexic." These youngsters appeared brighter than they were because they were able to read. However, they did not understand much of what they read. In fact, their good visual memory created something of a problem for these particular pupils, since their parents and teachers often expected more from them than they were able to accomplish. When the expected achievement was not forthcoming, the children were frequently regarded as "lazy." These "hyperlexic" pupils read

1

mostly by rote and had difficulty integrating what they read; they were usually unable to generalize from one lesson to another.

The third group of children who required five or more years of special education were of average mental ability but had severe learning disabilities. Among other problems, these youngsters suffered from a marked memory deficit for sound and symbol integration and sequencing. In consequence, they had very serious reading and writing difficulties. Reading and writing involve both visual and auditory memory for letters and sounds and for the sequences of sounds and symbols (Johnson and Myklebust, 1967, p. 150). Many of these youngsters forgot what they learned within a day or two.

It was interesting to note that the characteristic WISC (Wechsler, 1949) Subtest score pattern of this group of children, with severe learning disabilities, was quite similar to the WISC Subtest pattern of a group of pupils with specific learning problems, described by Ackerman et al. (1971), and of underachieving boys, studied by Jenkin et al. (1964). All three groups of youngsters had exceptionally low scores on the Information, Arithmetic, Digit Span, and Coding Subtests. These four WISC Subtests are all related to memory and recall: The Information Subtest involves long-term memory for facts and figures; the Arithmetic Subtest requires the ability to process and recall auditory instructions; the Digit Span Subtest assesses a child's ability to process, sequence, and remember auditorily presented digit sequences, whereas a good score on the Coding Subtest depends on the ability to memorize and reproduce from recall visual symbols at great speed.

The fourth group of long-term, learning-disabled pupils exhibited a variety of problems, the most significant of which were poor inner control and emotional and behavior disorders. Most of these children also showed a large discrepancy between their WISC Verbal IQ and Performance IQ scores. Sometimes the Verbal IQ scores were higher than the Performance IQ scores, whereas at other times the Performance IQ scores were the higher ones. Many of the youngsters had serious problems with intersensory integration.

Thus, it was shown that all four groups of long-term special class pupils had difficulties in the area of intersensory integration, sequencing, and recall. These problems were obviously not the only difficulties the youngsters had, but they contributed greatly to the pupils' lack of academic progress. A meaningful diagnosis of learning difficulties in schoolchildren should, therefore, include an evaluation of the children's functioning in integration, sequencing, and recall.

A number of other investigators have reported a significant relationship between memory for sequences of symbols and reading achievement. They include Johnson and Myklebust, 1967; Linder and Fillmer, 1970; Rose, 1958; Rudisil, 1956; Samuels and Anderson, 1973; and Sperling, 1960. It was also demonstrated that good or average readers score significantly higher on memory span tests than children with serious reading problems (Alwitt, 1963; Beery, 1967; Birch and Belmont, 1964; Farnham-Diggory and Gregg, 1974; Guthrie and Goldberg, 1972; Meeker, 1966; Spring, 1976; Wakefield, 1973).

What is the best way to evaluate children's intersensory integration,

sequencing, and recall without having to go through lengthy and compli-
cated testing procedures? For several years I searched in vain for a brief,
easy to administer, standardized test for schoolchildren that would give me
the information which I needed. Several memory tests for children are
available, but most of them deal with memory for designs rather than with
the recall of letters or digits. They do not include both sounds and symbols and
are directly related to school achievement. Reading and writing involve, of
course, the integration of sounds and symbols. The Stanford-Binet Intelligence Scale (Terman and Merrill, 1960), the Wechsler Intelligence Scale for
Children (Wechsler, 1949, 1974), and the Illinois Test of Psycholinguistic
Ability (Kirk et al., 1968) all include subtests of auditory sequencing and
memory and tests of visual memory, but none of them measures children's
ability for cross-modal sensory integration and recall.

A survey of the literature reveals numerous studies that involve the
memory span test performance of children. These studies were all concerned
with the immediate recall of information from short-term memory (STM)
only. Learning and school achievement require both STM and long-term
memory (LTM). Klatzky (1975, p. 229) describes STM very appropriately as
"working memory," the immediate, active component of memory in the
acquisition and processing of new information that is eventually transferred
to the dynamic storage of the LTM. If the STM malfunctions, the LTM will
also be impaired since the vital link between incoming information and
permanent storage is damaged. But the opposite is not necessarily true. Good
STM will not assure that a child will also have good LTM. Both STM and
LTM affect school achievement. But the evaluation of the children in clinical
or school settings is usually limited to one or two brief testing sessions and
observation periods, and most practicing psychologists or diagnosticians
limit their assessment mainly to children's STM. We are therefore primarily
concerned with STM.

STM can be measured in many different ways by means of memory span
tests. On Table 1 are listed the authors of memory span studies with children, the nature of stimuli used, the mode of presentation, and the mode of
response. Some of the studies used auditory stimuli; these involved digits
(Bridgeman and Buttram, 1975; Finch et al., 1976; Nalven, 1967; Senf, 1969),
words (Wachs, 1969), or taps (Birch and Belmont, 1964; Kahn and Birch,
1968). Other studies employed visual stimuli including digits (Alwitt, 1963),
letterlike forms (Samuels and Anderson, 1973), line drawings (London and
Robinson, 1968), and pictures (Leslie, 1975). Several investigators used both
auditory and visual stimuli (Beery, 1967; Farnham-Diggory and Gregg, 1974;
Lindner and Fillmer, 1970; Murray and Roberts, 1968; Rudel and Teuber,
1971). The subjects responded to the stimuli either verbally, in writing, or by
pointing to one of several alternative answers.

About half of the studies, listed on Table 1, involve intrasensory integration, whereas the other half involve intersensory integration. In the studies
with intrasensory integration the stimuli and the responses are both given in
the same sense modality, e.g., auditory presentation of digits and oral recall,
or visual presentation of digits and visual or written recall. Intersensory
integration involves the integration of two different sense modalities, e.g.,

Table 1.

Memory Span Studies with Children

Authors	Stimuli	Mode of Presentation	Mode of Response
Nalven (1967)	digits	aural	oral
Bridgeman & Buttram (1975)	digits	aural	oral
Finch et al. (1976)	digits	aural	oral
Birch & Belmont (1964)	taps	aural	visual
Kahn & Birch (1968)	taps	aural	visual
Wachs (1969)	words	aural	written
Alwitt (1963)	digits	visual	oral
Leslie (1975)	pictures	visual	oral
London & Robinson (1968)	line drawings	visual	visual
Samuels & Anderson (1973)	letterlike figures	visual	visual
Beery (1967)	taps	aural	visual
	code	visual	oral
Murray & Roberts (1968)	digits	aural	written
	letters, digits, pictures	visual	written
Farnham-Diggory & Gregg (1974)	letters	aural	oral
	letters	visual	oral
Lindner & Fillmer (1970)	digits,	aural	oral
	objects,	visual	oral
	colors	aural/visual	oral
Senf (1969)	digits	aural/visual	oral
Rudel & Teuber (1971)	taps	aural	aural
	taps	aural	visual
	visual code	visual	aural
	visual code	visual	visual

auditory presentation of digits and written recall, or visual presentation of digits and oral recall. The studies under discussion include examples of both visual and auditory intrasensory integration and intersensory integration.

In most of the studies only one type of integration was required of the subjects; there were, however, four exceptions. Murray and Roberts (1968) used both auditory-written and visual-written integration, that is, both intersensory and intrasensory integration. Senf (1969) and Lindner and Fillmer (1970) presented both auditory and visual stimuli separately as well as simultaneously, but all responses were oral.

Rudel and Teuber (1971) used Birch and Belmont's method of taps and visual codes as stimuli in two of their experiments. They asked their subjects to respond both visually and orally to aural taps and visual codes; that is, the children performed aural-oral, aural-visual, visual-oral, and visual-visual integrations. The study involved both intrasensory and intersensory integration in two different sense modalities. This was exactly the type of STM test I had hoped to find for use as a clinical instrument for schoolchildren. But Rudel and Teuber's stimuli of taps and visual codes were only incidentally related to school achievement. I was looking for a test that would be more closely related to reading, spelling, and arithmetic, and that would measure the mental processes involved in these basic skills.

Since I was unable to discover a test that met all of my criteria, I decided to develop my own test of integration, sequencing, and recall for school-age children. As stimuli I selected digits. I called the new test the Visual Aural Digit Span Test, or VADS Test to emphasize the integrational aspect. The use of digits rather than letters as stimuli was quite deliberate and carefully considered.

Reading and spelling depend on the ability to sequence and to recall letter constellations and specific sound-symbol associations. It stands to reason, therefore, that letters would be the ideal stimuli for a diagnostic test of learning problems. Indeed, Wakefield (1973) showed that average readers have better visual memory for letters than poor readers. But just because letters are so closely related to school achievement they also tend to acquire strong emotional connotations for children who have problems with reading and spelling. For pupils with learning difficulties, letters are often associated with failure and are, therefore, anything but neutral symbols. A child who cannot read and who cannot remember whether a given letter is called a *b* or a *d*, or whether the letter he is perceiving correctly is labeled *m* or *n*, tends to get anxious when he is asked to reproduce letter series from memory. And furthermore, it would be difficult to determine if failure to reproduce letter sequences correctly resulted from a youngster's problems with the labeling of letters or from the inability to remember and to reproduce the letters in the correct order. It was also found that pupils tried to read letters and tried to attach meaning to them when letters were used as stimuli. Some children attempt to form syllables or nonsense words from letter stimuli in an effort to remember them better. All of these reasons spoke against the selection of letters as stimuli for the new memory span test.

The use of digits as stimuli in a memory span test, on the other hand, has several advantages. There are only nine digits, not counting 0, as compared to 26 letters. Most school-age children are able to read and write the digits from 1 to 9 long before they have mastered all 26 letters. Digits are also symbols that are used in schoolwork, but they are much less anxiety provoking than letters, especially for children with learning disabilities. With these considerations in mind, I selected the digits from 1 to 9 as stimuli for the VADS Test.

INTRODUCTION: SUMMARY

Learning problems in schoolchildren result from the combination and interaction of many different causes. Learning-disabled children, requiring long-term special education, appear to have particular difficulty with intersensory integration, sequencing, and recall. Therefore, it is important to assess these factors when diagnosing learning disabilities in children. A survey of the literature failed to reveal a brief, easy to administer, standardized test of intersensory integration and short-term memory for school-age children. To fill this need, I developed the Visual Aural Digit Span Test, or VADS Test. The VADS Test uses the digits 1 to 9 for stimuli.

Chapter 2

Anxiety and Memory Span Tests

In clinical psychology the Digit Span Test had been traditionally considered a measure of anxiety (Cattell and Scheier, 1961, Wechsler, 1958). Over the years I have read numerous psychological reports that claimed that a youngster with serious learning or behavior problems scored markedly lower on the WISC Digit Span Subtest because of "severe anxiety." Most reports showed indeed that the child in question was an anxious youngster, yet there was no clear indication that the low score on the Digit Span Test was necessarily caused by the child's anxiety. The child's poor performance on the Digit Span Test could have evoked the anxiety or the anxiety and the low Digit Span scores could have coexisted without any causal relationship between them. Perhaps both the low scores and the anxiety resulted from an unidentified third factor. It seems, therefore, important to explore more fully the relationship between anxiety and Digit Span Test performance of children, for if memory span tests primarily measure anxiety, then their value as diagnostic tests for learning problems is questionable.

To begin with *anxiety* is a very ambiguous concept lacking a precise definition. There is no single factor of generalized anxiety. The consensus seems to be that anxiety is multidimensional. Cattell and Scheier (1961) differentiated between a transitory *anxiety state* and a more stable *anxiety condition.* Spielberger (1966) defined Anxiety State or A-State as a "subjective feeling of apprehension and concern and heightened autonomic nervous system acuity"; Anxiety State is transitory. Anxiety Trait or A-Trait is a stable condition that involves anxiety proneness and a "disposition to respond with high levels of Anxiety State under stressful circumstances."

The Taylor Manifest Anxiety Scale (Taylor, 1953) is frequently used to measure Anxiety Trait. A survey of the literature revealed a number of studies using both the Taylor Manifest Anxiety Scale and Digit Span tests. Unfortunately, most of these studies involve adults rather than children as subjects, yet the findings are of interest.

Matarazzo (1955) and Jackson and Bloomberg (1958), working with adult psychiatric patients, and Hodges and Spielberg (1969) and Walker and Spence (1966), testing college students, all failed to find a significant relationship between performance on the Taylor Manifest Anxiety Scale and Digit Span scores. Only Colvin et al. (1955) reported a significant correlation between the two measures for college students. It would appear, therefore, that the Taylor Manifest Anxiety Scale and the Digit Span Test are associated with different factors that may or may not be present simultaneously.

Research findings suggest that the Taylor Manifest Anxiety Scale measures, as claimed, mainly Anxiety Trait or anxiety proneness in adults

(Hodges and Spielberg, 1969; Jackson and Bloomberg, 1958; Matarazzo, 1955; Walker and Spence, 1964); whereas induced Anxiety State in college students seems to be related to a significant decrement on the Digit Span Test (Griffiths, 1958; Hodges and Spielberg, 1969; Moldowsky and Moldowsky, 1952; Pyke and Agnew, 1963; Walker and Spence, 1964).

Hodges and Spielberg hypothesize that college students develop the Anxiety State in response to their poor performance on the Digit Span Test. In other words, the Anxiety State is a response of the students to their own deteriorating performance rather than a reaction to the experimenter's instructions, which then in turn decreases their performance on the Digit Span Test further. Hodges and Spielberg's hypothesis concurs with my own observation and experience with children.

More recently, Finch et al. (1974) factor analyzed the performance of 245 children on the Children Manifest Anxiety Scale, or CMAS (Castanada et al., 1956). The CMAS was individually administered under conditions of no stress. The investigators found that anxiety was multidimensional; three distinct factors were identified that were specifically related to anxiety. These were interpreted as Factor I, Anxiety: Worry and Oversensitivity; Factor II, Anxiety: Physiological; and Factor III, Anxiety: Concentration. Anxiety: Worry and Oversensitivity is shown by children whose anxiety takes the form of worry and effects their thought processes; Anxiety: Physiological is shown by children who respond to anxiety with somatic manifestations; whereas Anxiety: Concentration is shown by youngsters whose anxiety interferes with their ability to concentrate and to perform tasks.

Finch et al. (1976) also explored the relationship of the test scores of 38 emotionally disturbed children on the CMAS and on the auditory sequential memory section (digit span) of the Illinois Test of Psycholinguistic Ability (Kirk et al., 1968). All the children were of average or better mental ability; their age mean was 10 years 9 months. The results failed to show any significant relationship between the Digit Span Test scores and high or low performance on the Total CMAS, or on Factor I, Anxiety: Worry and Oversensitivity or Factor II, Anxiety: Physiological. But youngsters who scored high on Factor III, Anxiety: Concentration did significantly less well (F 10.86, $p < .01$) on the Digit Span Test than children who scored low on Factor III, Anxiety: Concentration.

It stands to reason that a good performance on the Digit Span Test requires concentration. Children with poor concentration can be expected to have difficulty with the recall of a series of digits. But the study of Finch et al. leaves several questions unanswered. Did the youngsters in the study have difficulty concentrating because they were anxious, or were they anxious because they were distractible and had a short attention span and difficulty concentrating? Also, was there any relationship between the children's IQ scores and Factor III, Anxiety: Concentration?

Nalven (1967) correlated the WISC Digit Span scores of emotionally disturbed children with Distractibility, as measured on the Devereux Child Behavior Rating Scale. Distractibility would most certainly influence a child's ability to concentrate. Nalven obtained a significant correlation ($p <$

.05) between the two measures, however, when the Full Scale IQ was partialed out the relationship between the two test scores was no longer significant.

On the basis of my experience, I concur with Hodges and Spielberg that poor concentration leads to poor performance on the Digit Span Test; children's awareness of their poor Digit Span Test scores results then in Anxiety State. Therefore, Anxiety State is usually secondary to problems with concentration and to low Digit Span scores. Only in exceptional cases will a child be in such an acute emotional crisis that he is too anxious to concentrate and is unable to recall digit sequences. Under such circumstances the youngster will be most likely unable to perform any formal task and testing becomes meaningless. In such an event, testing should be discontinued until some other time.

As was previously indicated, many pupils with learning problems obtain poor scores on memory span tests even when they are tested individually in nonstressful situations, and when they are relaxed and at ease. The low test scores seem to reflect most often poor ability in sequencing and recall of series of symbols rather than anxiety. Research findings and my clinical experience convinced me that memory span tests are primarily tests of intersensory integration and short-term memory, and only secondarily measures of anxiety.

If anxiety plays only a subordinated role in memory test performance, what other factors account then for children's difficulties with the recall of symbol sequences? A number of explanations, in addition to anxiety, have been suggested for poor memory span performances. Many types of memory disturbances, including deficits in memory span and immediate and delayed recall, have been attributed to Central Nervous System dysfunction (Johnson and Myklebust, 1967, p. 150) or brain injury (Birch and Belmont, 1965 a). Other specific causes have been mentioned: Deficits in "trace function" or short-term memory (Baumeister et al., 1963); poor visual memory and difficulty in sequencing (Senf, 1969); problems with intrasensory integration and with crossmodal (aural-visual) integration (Birch and Belmont, 1965 a; Senf 1969); failure to rehearse digits and to use verbal mediation (Senf, 1969); failure to reorganize or chunk digits (Miller, 1956; Senf, 1969); developmental lag (Lyle and Goyen, 1968); failure to pay attention to the entire field and processing of only part of the presented digits, and difficulty in associating memory and verbal response (Alwitt, 1963); limit in capability of holding information in memory (Alwitt, 1963; Mahoney, 1972; Spitz, 1973).

It would appear, therefore, that several different factors contribute to children's performance on memory span tests. There is an agreement among investigators that memory span tests measure intersensory and intrasensory integration, sequencing, and recall. Memory span tests are thus well qualified to serve as diagnostic instruments for learning problems associated with integration and short-tem memory problems. The Visual Aural Digit Span Test is such a test.

The following chapters describe the Visual Aural Digit Span Test in detail and present normative data, research findings, case histories, and the application of the test in a screening battery for school beginners.

ANXIETY AND MEMORY SPAN TESTS: SUMMARY

A survey of the literature shows a consensus that anxiety is multidimensional. One can distinguish between a relatively stable Anxiety Trait and a temporary Anxiety State response. Anxiety Trait can be measured with the Taylor Manifest Anxiety Scale; Anxiety Trait is not related to memory span test performance. Anxiety State correlates positively with memory span test performance, but the nature of this relationship is unclear.

Based on my experience, I maintain that Anxiety State is usually secondary to poor concentration and poor memory span test performance. Memory span tests, including the Visual Aural Digit Span Test, are mainly measures of intersensory integration, sequencing, and recall; as such they are well suited to serve as diagnostic instruments for learning disabilities in schoolchildren.

Chapter 3

Description of the Visual Aural Digit Span Test

The Visual Aural Digit Span Test, or VADS Test hereafter, was designed to serve as a diagnostic instrument for children age 5½ to 12, or for end-of-kindergarten pupils to sixth graders. At the beginning of kindergarten children are not yet able to cope with the VADS Test.

The VADS Test consists of four Subtests. The first of these is the easiest one. It requires merely the oral repetition of spoken or aurally presented series of digits. The second Subtest requires that a youngster be able to read printed digits and can say their names. The third Subtest involves the hearing and writing of digits from memory, whereas the fourth Subtest demands the reading and writing of digits. Most children learn to read digits and can copy them before they are able to write them from memory. Thus, the four VADS Subtests are arranged in the order in which children acquire the necessary skills to perform them. Any youngster who can hear and say digits can take the first VADS Subtest. A child who can read digits can finish the second Subtest also, even if he cannot as yet write digits. But the complete administration of the VADS Test presupposes that the youngsters are able to read and write digits. The test is thus not appropriate for pupils before the age of 5½ or 6 years, since younger children cannot be expected to possess the necessary skills needed to perform the VADS Test in its entirety.

The four VADS Subtests involve the reproduction of two-digit to seven-digit series. No longer digit sequences are used because, as Miller (1956) pointed out in his paper on the "magic number seven," our immediate memory is limited to seven items or "chunks of information." Simon (1974) also found that the short-term memory can store and recall roughly seven "chunks." Spitz (1972) made a survey of studies on immediate memory for visually and auditorily presented digits. He found that the "channel capacity" (which was defined as more than 90% correct recall) for average adolescents and adults varies remarkably little; it was six, plus or minus one. Thus, there seemed little value in asking children to recall more than seven-digit sequences on the VADS Test. Any youngster who is able to master a seven-digit sequence possesses a fully developed, well-functioning short-term memory.

The four VADS Subtests are shown on Plate 1. The digit sequences used as stimuli for the four VADS Subtests are to be found on the 26 VADS Test stimulus cards (Koppitz, 1977 a). The four VADS Subtests are as follows:

I. *Aural-Oral Subtest* (A-O): This Subtest involves the aural presentation of the series of digits shown on Card 1-1 and their oral recall. This

VISUAL AURAL DIGIT SPAN TEST

(VADS TEST)

1st Subtest
AURAL-ORAL

(A–O)

3rd Subtest
AURAL-WRITTEN

(A–W)

2nd Subtest
VISUAL-ORAL

(V–O)

4th Subtest
VISUAL-WRITTEN

(V–W)

Plate 1.

Subtest is similar to the traditional Digit Span Test on the Stanford-Binet Intelligence Test and on the WISC. It shows how well a youngster can process and repeat aural stimuli in the correct order. The Subtest measures the integration of auditory perception, sequencing, and recall.

II. *Visual-Oral Subtest* (V-O): This Subtest involves the visual presentation of the series of digits shown on Cards 2-A to 2-10 and their oral recall in the correct order. This Subtest shows how well a pupil can process visual stimuli and can recall them orally; that is, it measures visual-oral integration and memory. A similar process is required when reading aloud from a printed page.

III. *Aural-Written Subtest* (A-W): This Subtest involves the aural presentation of the series of digits shown on Card 3-1 and their written reproduction. An Aural-Written Subtest shows how well a pupil can process, sequence, and recall auditory stimuli and translate them into written symbols. The Subtest measures auditory-visual integration and memory. A similar process is involved when writing words or sentences from dictation.

IV. *Visual-Written Subtest* (V-W): This Subtest involves the visual presentation of the series of digits shown on Cards 4-A to 4-10 and their written reproduction from memory. The Visual-Written Subtest shows how well a pupil can process, sequence, and recall visual stimuli; that is, it measures the intrasensory integration of visual input and written expression. This process is involved when a youngster is asked to copy from memory what he has seen.

ADMINISTRATION OF THE VADS TEST

Materials Needed

A set of 26 VADS Test stimulus cards (Koppitz, 1977 a), a blank sheet of paper, size 8½ × 11 inches, and a No. 2 pencil with an eraser for the pupil, and a pencil, a VADS Test scoring sheet (Koppitz, 1977 b), and a wristwatch with a second hand, or a stopwatch or any other inconspicuous timing device, for the examiner.

Procedure

After the child is comfortably seated at a table or desk, show him the pack of VADS Test cards. Depending on the child's age, say: "Here are some cards with numbers on them; we are going to play a game with them," or "Here are some cards with numbers on them; I want to see how well you can remember numbers." Then proceed with the first Subtest. Answer any questions the child may have in a noncommittal manner. Observe the child during the test administration and note down not only his responses but also his attitude and behavior.

I. *Aural-Oral* (Card 1-1): Say, "First I am going to say some numbers to you, and when I am finished I want you to say them after me." *Read off digits at the rate of one per second* (Practice reading digits beforehand until you are able to read them in an even rhythm without any grouping of the digits). With 5½- to 6-year-old children start with the first three-digit sequence. If the child fails the first three-digit sequence, give him the second three-digit sequence. If he fails both trials with the three-digit sequences, give him one or both two-digit sequences until he passes them, then discontinue this Subtest. If the child repeats one of the three-digit sequences correctly, go on to the first four-digit sequence, and so on. Discontinue this Subtest when the child fails both trials of any one digit series.

With 7- to 9-year-old children, or with older retarded youngsters, start with the first four-digit sequences. If the child fails both four-digit sequences give him one or both three-digit sequences until he repeats a sequence correctly, then discontinue this Subtest. If he passes one of the four-digit sequences, go on to the five-digit sequences. Continue until the child misses both trials of a given sequence of digits. With children age 10 or older, who are not retarded, start with the first five-digit sequence and proceed in the same manner.

Note on the scoring sheet the sequences passed or missed and whether failure resulted from incorrect sequencing of digits, from omissions or additions of digits, or whether the child had a total lack of recall; note whether the child grouped digits as he repeated them.

II. *Visual-Oral* (Cards 2-A to 2-10): This Subtest presupposes that the child is able to read digits. In case of doubt, have the child read out loud the digits on Card 2-10 as this card contains all digits from 3 to 9. If the child is unable to read most digits, omit this Subtest as well as the Visual-Written Subtest.

If the child confuses 6 and 9, but can read the other digits correctly, proceed with the Subtest but make allowance for the confusion as long as it is consistent. In order to assertain whether a youngster is actually repeating what he reads, it is recommended that school beginners and retarded youngsters be asked to read all digit sequences out loud rather than silently.

If the child can read digits, say: "This time I am going to show you some numbers and I want you to say them *after* I have taken the card away. There is no hurry, you may look at the card as long as I show it to you." Show the card for 10 seconds, then remove the card and have child say the digits one by one. If child says "six hundred-eighty-three" for Card 2-1, say: "yes, that is what it says, but I would like you to say each number separately like this, 6-8-3."

With 5½- and 6-year-old children, begin with the first three-digit sequence on Card 2-1. If the child fails to say this sequence correctly show him Card 2-2 with the second three-digit series. If the child misses both trials with the three-digit sequences, show him the two-digit series on Card 2-A, and Card 2-B if needed, then discontinue this Subtest. If the child repeats either the first or the second three-digit sequence without error show him Card 2-3 with the first four-digit series, and so on. Discontinue this Subtest when the child misses both trials of a given digit sequence.

The same procedure is followed with older children, but with 7- to 9-

year-old youngsters, or with older retarded children, start with the first four-digit sequence (Card 2-3); with children age 10 or older, who are not retarded, start with the first five-digit sequence (Card 2-5).

III. *Aural-Written* (Card 3-1): Give the child the blank sheet of paper and the pencil with an eraser. This Subtest presupposes that the child can write digits. With 5½- to 6-year-old pupils, or in case of doubt with older children, have them write the digits from 1 to 9 across the top of the paper. If the digits are clearly recognizable, even though some may be written incorrectly or reversed, as shown in Plate 2,* continue the Subtest. Note difficulties with the writing of digits on the scoring sheet. If the child is unable to make recognizable digits (see Plate 3), or if he does not know the names of the digits he draws, then omit this Subtest and the Visual-Written Subtest.

If the child is able to write the digits from 1 to 9 say: "Now I am going to say some numbers and I want you to write them down *after* I have finished saying them." Say the digits at the rate of one per second. With 5½- to 7-year-old, children and with retarded pupils, begin the first 3-digit sequence; with 8- to 12-year olds, who are not retarded, begin with the first 4-digit sequence. Proceed as in Subtests I and II; if the child reproduces one series of digits correctly go on to the next higher series of digits. If the child fails both trials of the first series of digits presented, go back to the preceding lower series of digits until the youngster is able to reproduce a sequence of digits correctly. Then discontinue this Subtest.

IV. *Visual-Written* (Cards 4-A to 4-10): This Subtest presupposes that the child can read and write digits. If the child is unable to do so, omit this Subtest. If the child can read and write digits, say: "This time I will show you some numbers and *after* I take the card away I want you to write them down." *Show each card for 10 seconds.*

With 5½- to 6-year-old children, or with retarded youngsters, begin with the first three-digit sequence (Card 4-1); with 7- to 9-year-olds begin with the first four-digit sequence (Card 4-3) and with children age 10 or older start with the first five-digit sequence (Card 4-5). Proceed as in the other Subtests. Discontinue after failure on both trials of a given digit sequence.

Some very young or impulsive children may have difficulty waiting for 10 seconds before responding to the stimulus cards. Such youngsters should be reminded that there is no hurry and that they should wait until the card is removed. If they persist in reproducing the digits before the 10 seconds are up, and if their response is incorrect, then something like the following statement may be in order: "You were too much in a hurry that time and did not get the numbers quite right. This time try and slow down, take your time and see if you can get the numbers exactly right."

After completion of the VADS Test ask the child to write his name on the VADS Test protocol so you can obtain a sample of his handwriting as well.

---

*All plates have been reduced 45% from their original size.

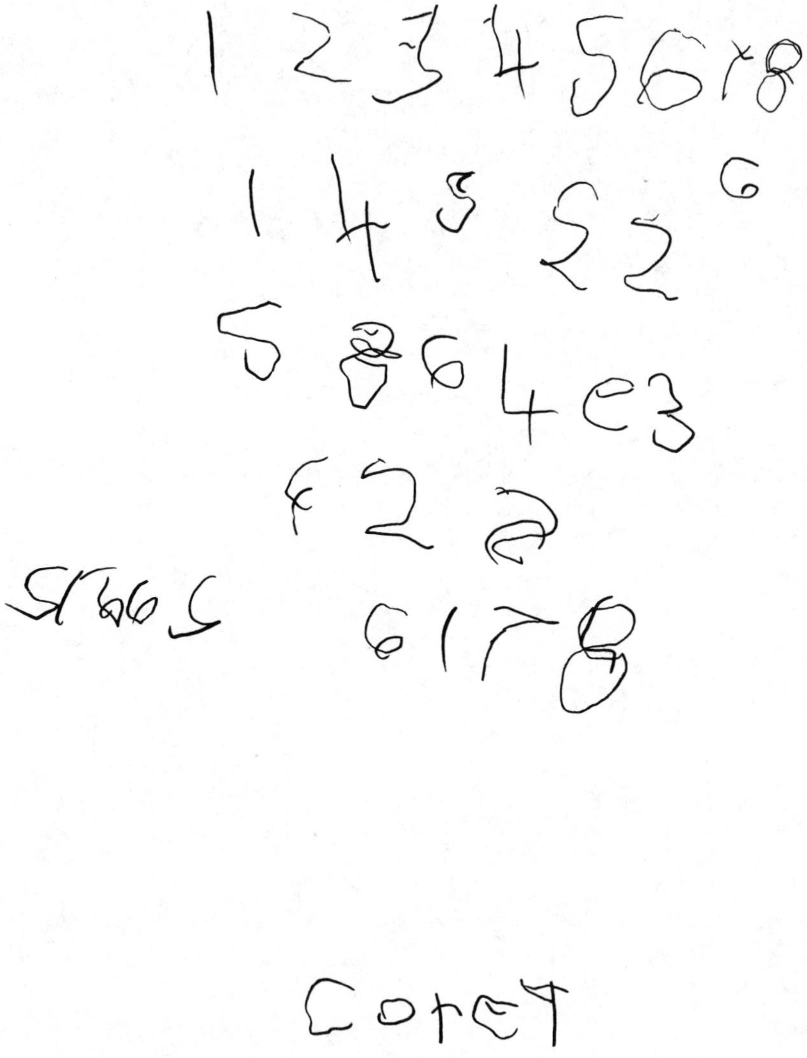

1 2 3 4 5 6 8

1 4 5 5 2 6

5 8 6 4 e3

5 2 a

5965 6 1 7 8

Corey

Plate 2. Corey, C.A. 6–0.

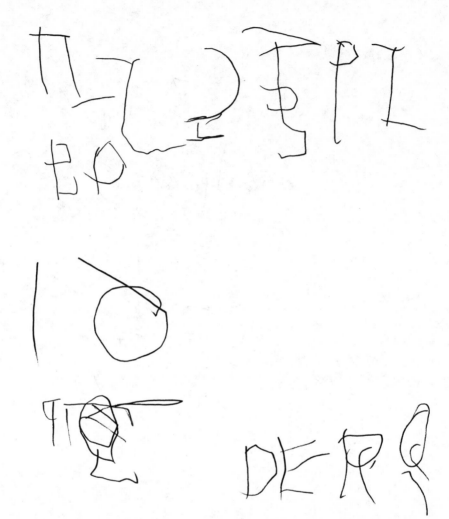

Plate 3. Derrick, C.A. 6–4.

Chapter 4

Interpretation of the VADS Test

The VADS Test, like most other psychological tests, should be interpreted in at least three different ways (Koppitz, 1975a, p. 5), so as to obtain the most information and value from it. A great deal more can be derived from the VADS Test than merely test scores. A youngster's attitudes and behavior while taking the test are also of considerable diagnostic significance, and of equal importance is the quality of the test protocol. Finally there are the VADS Test scores, which can also be analyzed in several different ways.

BEHAVIOR OBSERVATIONS

A child's attitude toward a task will greatly influence his test performance. Therefore it is essential to determine whether the youngster taking the test is motivated and cooperative, or whether he is resistant or indifferent. Is the child at ease and does he put forth effort, or is he tense and lacking in self-confidence? Does the youngster have a need to succeed? Is he ambitious and does he want to know if he did better than other children? Does the pupil exclaim: "This is easy, I will get them all right!", only to get anxious and discouraged when he fails to reproduce a digit sequence correctly? A child who gives up and stops trying when he meets with frustration will also stop doing his work in school when he experiences failure.

How impulsive is the youngster? How good are his inner controls? The VADS Test requires concentration and attention; some children find it hard to concentrate for any length of time. These impulsive youngsters begin to repeat digits before the examiner has finished saying the last ones, or they start writing digits before the examiner has exposed the test cards for 10 seconds. Some children grab hold of the test cards and turn them face down rather than wait for the signal to start writing. Such pupils will also begin to answer questions or assignments in class before they have found out what they are required to do.

Some youngsters have a short attention span; they may start the VADS Test with great enthusiasm and do very well at first, but before long they tire and are no longer able to concentrate as well as before. These same children often have poor intersensory integration and are impulsive. They have to exert more energy than most pupils to perform tasks of mental concentration. In consequence, these children tend to fatigue quickly and start failing; they usually require a brief period of rest or change of activity before they can resume their optimal performance. Youngsters who alternately pass and fail digit sequences on the VADS Test also tend to function unevenly in school;

17

they may find it very difficult to concentrate for a whole period on one assignment. But if given extra time to complete the assignment and a few brief breaks during the study period, then they usually do satisfactory work.

How good is a child's frustration tolerance? Younger children invariably miss some of the digit series on the VADS Test. The way they react to such failures is often characteristic of their way of coping with failure in the classroom. Some children get disgusted when they cannot recall a digit or two. They may scribble over their work impulsively, as is shown on Plate 4. A few youngsters will even try to destroy the protocol. Some pupils become anxious and tense when they cannot complete a digit sequence and look to the examiner for help and reassurance. Others can say in a matter-of-fact way that they do not remember a digit and are able to continue the test without much upset. It is interesting to note how some youngsters will guess without hesitation, when they cannot recall a digit, whereas others are unwilling to guess or to take chances. The latter are the ones who will sit in class and do nothing when they are unsure about an answer; they are too anxious and shy to ask for help, and too insecure to guess. Very young and very dull children are often quite unaware of their errors on the VADS Test.

Even in a quiet office or testing room there are sometimes unavoidable distractions. The VADS Test performance provides a good opportunity for the examiner to observe the child's degree of distractibility and his restlessness. Is the youngster bothered by noise in the hall or activity outside the window? Can the child sit still or is he hyperactive? Does he wiggle in his seat or rock on the chair? Is his body in constant motion? Does he grab and touch everything in sight? Does he display nervous mannerisms? Does he tap his fingers or pencil? Does he have an eye tic or bite his fingernails? Does he twist his hair or suck his thumb? Does he ask to go to the bathroom every few minutes?

How good is a pupil's coordination? Does he hold the pencil awkwardly? Is he right-handed or left-handed or ambidextrous? Does the child hold the VADS Test cards close to his face when looking at the digits or does he hold them far away from him? Does he close one eye or turn his head while reading the digits? Does he have a visual problem? In the standardized administration of the VADS Test the examiner holds the test cards, but sometimes youngsters with visual problems need to hold the cards themselves at a given angle or distance in order to see the digits. It is also important to establish whether the child has glasses or not; many times pupils have glasses but will not wear them unless they are specifically told to do so. Occasionally a child will ask to have some of the VADS Test digit sequences repeated or show signs of having difficulty in hearing. Behavior of this type should be, of course, noted and further investigated.

Well-functioning children work with deliberate speed, neither too fast nor two slowly. Many impulsive children work very fast and carelessly both on the VADS Test and when doing their schoolwork. But others are extremely slow and careful in their execution of the VADS Test. Only observation of the youngster at work can tell whether the child is working slowly because he is hypoactive and lethargic, whether he is working slowly in an effort to control and overcome his impulsivity, or whether he is a

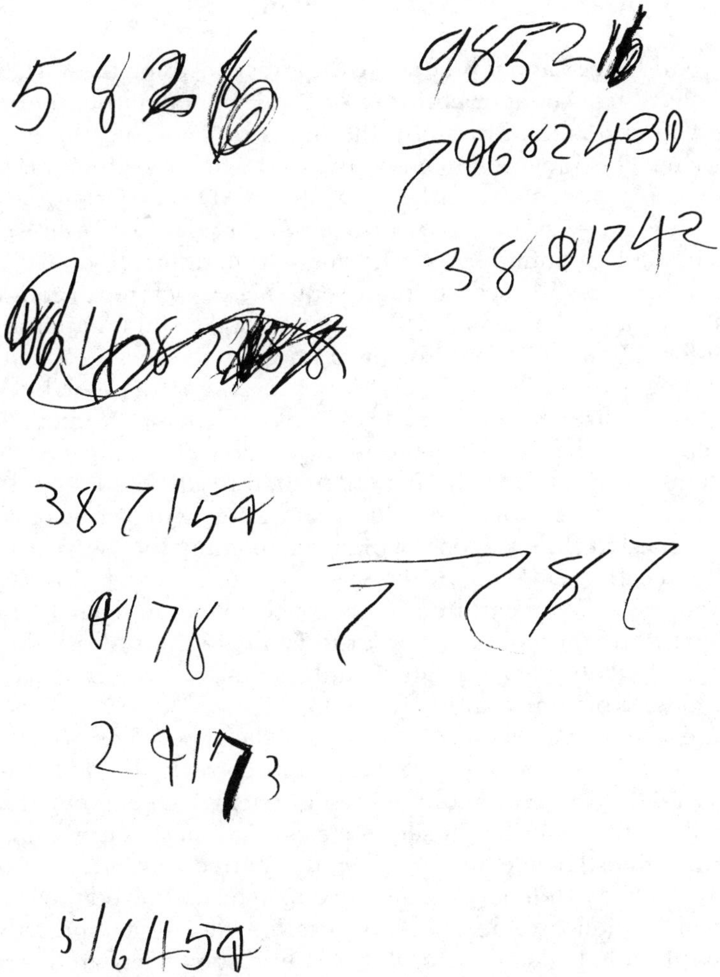

Plate 4. Fred, C.A. 10–8.

perfectionist who keeps on writing and rewriting digits until they are exactly
even and neat even though the child may forget some of the digits in the
process.

QUALITY OF TEST PERFORMANCE

The way children go about producing their responses on the VADS Test
can be very revealing. Younger children of good mental ability and older,
more mature youngsters tend to group the digits by twos and threes when
they repeat them. This process is commonly used when recalling telephone
numbers. When reproducing the digits 374697 (VADS Test Card 2-8), for
instance, the pupils may say 37-46-97 or 374-697, or possibly 37-469-7. For,
as Tulving (1966) has pointed out, the mere repetition of digits is not
sufficient for the successful recall of digit sequences; such recall requires a
"subjective organization" of them. Miller (1956) speaks of the importance of
"recoding" information by "chunking" it to improve the recall capacity.

The grouping of digits improves children's recall up to a point, but as the
chunks increase in size the memory for chunks decreases (Simon, 1974).
Thus, it was observed that some immature pupils do well on the VADS Test
when they chunk the digits by twos, but fail in their recall when they attempt
to group the digits by threes or fours. Many youngsters with serious learning
difficulties, or retarded children, do not organize or group the digits at all, but
instead try to recall them one by one. One would expect this type of
processing from very young children; however, when a pupil age 9 or older
makes no attempt to group digits in order to facilitate their recall, then the
youngster is most likely very immature and mentally limited, or has very
poor organizing and planning ability.

Great care should be taken to note down the type of errors children
make on the VADS Test. Do they repeat all digits correctly but in the wrong
order? That is, do they have difficulty with sequencing? One or two transpo-
sitions of digits on the longer digit sequences are not necessarily diagnostically significant. Koestler and Jenkins (1965) reported that one half of the
errors made by college students on a memory span test involved the transposition of visual sequences; the students recalled the digits correctly but
forgot their position in the sequence. But if a child shows repeated errors of
placement even in the easier four- and five-digit series, then he may have
specific problems with sequencing of sounds and symbols that would be, of
course, also reflected in his reading and spelling achievement.

Does a youngster remember only the first digits of a digit sequence and
have difficulty recalling the last ones? Or does a child remember only the last
digits while forgetting the first ones? These different types of errors are
closely related to problems in reading, spelling, and arithmetic. The child
who has difficulty with the sequencing of digits may also show problems
with the sequencing of letters and sounds; thus he may read "bluk" for
"bulk" or "slip" for "spill." The pupil who recalls only the first digits of a
sequence frequently shows the same tendency when reading; he may read
only the beginning of a word or sentence and then guess the rest. The

youngster who forgets the first digits of a sequence is also likely to forget part of the instructions given by the teacher, or he may fail to remember part of the process of long division.

Does a child have difficulty pronouncing the digits correctly? Does he display articulation or speech problems?

Does a youngster rehearse the digits spontaneously, either vocally or subvocally, as he tries to remember them? Spontaneous rehearsal occurs primarily with visually presented stimuli (Corballis and Loveless, 1967) and involves speech. According to Klatzky (1975, p. 68) items to be remembered are usually stored acoustically in the STM; however, rehearsal can also occur visually, but visual rehearsal is much slower and requires more time.

It was found that children who use verbal rehearsal on a memory task are more successful in recalling visual stimuli than youngsters who do not rehearse. The incidence of spontaneous verbal rehearsal increases significantly as children get older. Flavell et al. (1966) and Daehler et al. (1969) showed that kindergarten pupils do not use verbal rehearsal. At age 6 and 7 some pupils engage in spontaneous rehearsal routinely and use verbal mediation to aid them in recall, but many others do not, even though they possess the necessary linguistic ability to do so. Keeney et al. (1967) were able to teach the "nonrehearsers" how to use verbal mediation and rehearsal whereupon the youngsters' recall performance improved greatly and equaled that of the spontaneous "rehearsers." Yet, even after they had learned how to use verbal rehearsal the "nonrehearsers" chose not to employ this skill unless they were specifically asked to do so. Spontaneous verbal rehearsal did not occur regularly until the youngsters were in the fourth or fifth grade. Thus, it appears that spontaneous rehearsal by a young child is a sign of maturity and good mental ability, whereas the failure of older children to use spontaneous verbal mediation and rehearsal on a memory task may reveal specific learning difficulties or limited mental ability. In either case, youngsters who do not use such strategies spontaneously can evidently be taught to do so.

Brighter and older children often find ways to help them remember the digits on the VADS Test. Some youngsters not only repeat the digits to themselves but they also trace the digits in the air or on the table with a finger while they are hearing them. Some try to devise finger cues. The vocalization or subvocalization of digits is especially effective when children have to write the digits down; this method enables the youngsters to use both visual and auditory cues. It also provides valuable diagnostic clues.

Observation sometimes reveals that a pupil will *say* a sequence of digits correctly to himself only *to write* it down incorrectly. For example, he may say "*216*" but write *219*. If this happens consistently with the 6 and 9 only, then chances are that the youngster confuses the two digits and needs help in differentiating between them. But if this type of error is inconsistent and occurs with different digits, the youngster may have a problem with written expression.

It is not unusual for young children to omit or to add a digit when recalling a digit sequence. This type of error becomes only significant when older children persist in this pattern. A 10-year-old pupil who regularly omits digits may also omit steps when working a math problem or may leave out letters or words when reading.

Occasionally a child will reproduce one series of digits correctly and will then miss the following sequences because he repeats the same combination of digits over and over again, in other words, he perseverates on a given response. Perseveration occurs most often with young, insecure children with minimal brain dysfunction. Some of the youngsters are too rigid to be able to shift to new responses, whereas others try to repeat their initial success by repeating the same digit sequence, especially if they were praised for the first correct response. Perseveration and extreme rigidity interfere also grossly with school achievement.

Plate 5 shows the VADS Test record of Burt, age 11, a neurologically impaired youngster who suffered from a serious expressive disorder that affected both his speech and writing, and from perseveration. Burt was very cooperative and put forth effort during the administration of the VADS Test. On the Aural-Written Subtest he verbalized the digits as he wrote them. As can be seen on Plate 5, he wrote the three-digit sequence 532 correctly but continued the line of the 2 for an extra curve before he was able to stop himself. The same happened on the next digit series. Burt said and wrote the four-digit sequence correctly but this time both the 2 and the 6 were written with extra extensions and loops. Burt could not seem to control his hand while concentrating on the digits. Perseveration was carried to an extreme on the third row on Plate 5. Burt was unable to retain a five-digit sequence in his memory; he was aware of this and became quite anxious. He began writing the last digit, the 5, over and over again. He did not stop until he reached the edge of the paper. Burt looked rather embarrassed by his production and grinned sheepishly; he knew that what he had done was not correct but he just could not stop himself from doing it. The same pattern of perseveration was also apparent in his speech and in his schoolwork. On the Visual-Written Subtest, Burt also verbalized the digits as he wrote them down. He *said* 9-1-7-8 but *wrote* 9179, and he *said* 2-9-7-6-3 but wrote 29765. In both cases Burt was aware of his errors and corrected them spontaneously.

QUALITY OF TEST PERFORMANCE: SUMMARY

A child's approach to the VADS Test has considerable diagnostic significance. The recall of digit sequences is greatly aided when the digits are grouped into chunks and when they are verbally rehearsed. Brighter and older children tend to use these strategies spontaneously, but very young children and slow youngsters and pupils with learning disabilities usually fail to do so.

The types of errors that children make on the VADS Test often reflect problems that interfere with their reading and writing achievement. Such errors include problems with the sequencing of sounds and symbols, difficulty with the recall of the beginnings or endings of digit sequences or words, poor concentration and attention to only part of a digit sequence or word or instructions, disorders of written expression, and perseveration.

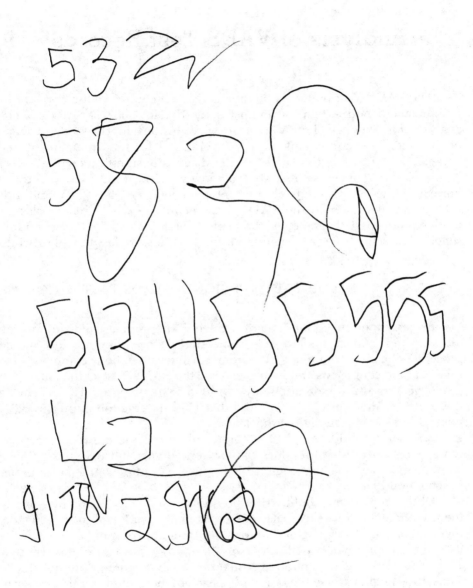

Plate 5. Burt. C.A. 11–0.

Chapter 5

Analysis of VADS Test Records

The VADS Test protocols provide a visual record of youngsters' ability to write and organize digits on an unstructured field. The test records can be analyzed for evidence of digit reversals or confusions, for the size and shape of the digits, for corrections and overwork, and for the arrangement and organization of the digits. To assess the diagnostic significance of a VADS Test record it is, of course, essential to know what the VADS Test records of normal public school pupils of different age levels look like. To obtain this information, I examined the VADS Test records of whole school classes, kindergarten to sixth grade, in three elementary schools and one middle school. The schools were located in middle- and lower-class neighborhoods.

REVERSALS AND DIGIT CONFUSION ON VADS TEST RECORDS

As any experienced kindergarten teacher knows, many 5½- and 6-year-old children confuse and reverse some digits since they are just in the process of learning numbers. In order to determine how common such reversals and confusions are, I administered the VADS Test, at the end of the school year, to 142 kindergarten pupils and to 58 first-graders. Table 2 shows the results of this study. It was found that 117 kindergarten pupils, or 82%, were able to write the digits from 1 to 9.

Another 17 children, or 12%, could only write the digits 1 to 5. Two others were only able to produce two or three digits, and six pupils, or 5%, were unable to write any recognizable digits. An example of the latter group is shown on Plate 3.

Of the pupils who could write the digits 1 to 9, only 20, or 14%, wrote them without any reversals whatsoever. As many as 21% of the youngsters reversed one or two digits; for example, they might reverse either the 3 or the 9, or they might reverse both the 3 and 9, or any other two digits. Another 21% of the kindergarten pupils reversed as many as three different digits. Thus, they might reverse the 6, 7, and 9; each of these digits might appear in reversal either once or more often on a single VADS Test record, yet each digit was counted only once as a reversal. More than one-fourth of the youngsters reversed four or more of the nine digits on the VADS Test record. Plate 6 shows the VADS Test record of Mark, age 5 years 8 months, with six reversals.

A comparison of the number of digit reversals on the VADS Test records of the kindergarten pupils and first-graders shows a significant difference

Table 2.

Digit Reversals or Less Than Nine Digits on VADS Test Records

	K Pupils (N 142)		First-Graders (N 58)	
	N	%	N	%
No reversals	20	14	45	78
One or two reversals	30	21	11	19
Three reversals	30	21	2	3
Four or more reversals	37	26	0	0
Digits 1 to 5 only	17	12	0	0
Less than five digits	2	1	0	0
No digits	6	5	0	0

between the two groups. All of the first-graders were able to write digits; 45 of them, or 78%, revealed no reversals. Of the first-graders 14% reversed one of the nine digits, 5% reversed two of the digits, and 3% reversed three digits.

Thus, it appears that the reversal of one, two, or three digits on the VADS Test records of kindergarten pupils is common, and presents no major reason for concern. However, when a 5½- or 6-year-old child persists in reversing more than three digits, after attending kindergarten for a year, then he may be immature for his age and may need some special assistance with the writing of digits. If, at the end of the first grade, a pupil still reverses digits then he may have perceptual problems or specific problems with directionality and visual-motor integration.

Most children enjoy taking the VADS Test, but it does require intense concentration and effort from the youngsters. Thus, pupils who ordinarily no longer reverse digits may reverse one or two digits on the VADS Test records while concentrating on the recall of the digit series. It is important to notice whether a child reverses a given digit only once under the pressure of the situation, or whether he reverses a digit consistently. If the reversals are consistent, then the youngster may have real problems with the direction of digits and may have not yet mastered the writing of numbers. If reversals occur only once on a digit, then this may merely signify that the writing of the digit is not yet entirely automatic, and that the child regressed temporarily while concentrating on the digit series, or that the youngster was tired.

Occasionally a pupil reverses not only individual digits but also the order of the digits. Plate 7 presents the VADS Test record of Michelle, age 6 years. When asked to write the digits from 1 to 9, she reversed the digits 3, 5, 7, and 9. On the Aural-Written and Visual-Written Subtests, Michelle reversed not only the digits but she also wrote from right to left, reversing the order of the digits. Instead of 532, Michelle wrote 534, beginning with the 4, then the 3, then the 5. Instead of 426 she wrote 624. But this time the digits appear correct since Michelle wrote again from right to left: 4-2-6.

Veronica was 6 years 4 months old when she produced the VADS Test record shown on Plate 8. She reversed the digits 3, 7, and 9, and wrote the digits 2, 5, and 6 upside down. Veronica had no difficulty matching digits;

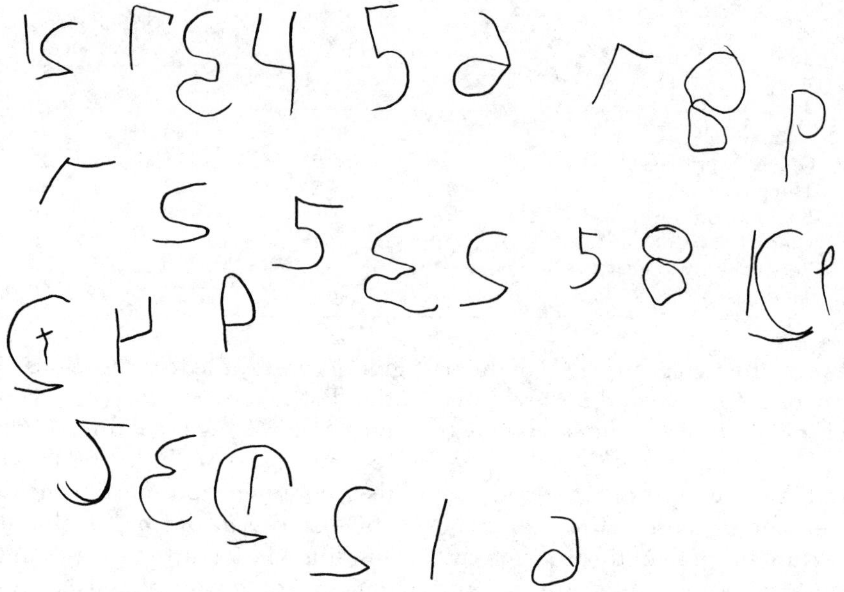

Reversals: 2, 3, 4, 6, 7, 9

Plate 6. Mark, C.A. 5–8.

12Ɛ4Ƨ6ΓØP 10 3̄1
Ɔ̄ 34ОPΓØ̄1
14 624
Ɔ̄О4Ɔ̄Ƨ

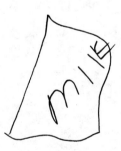

digit and sequence reversals

Plate 7. Michelle, C.A. 6–0.

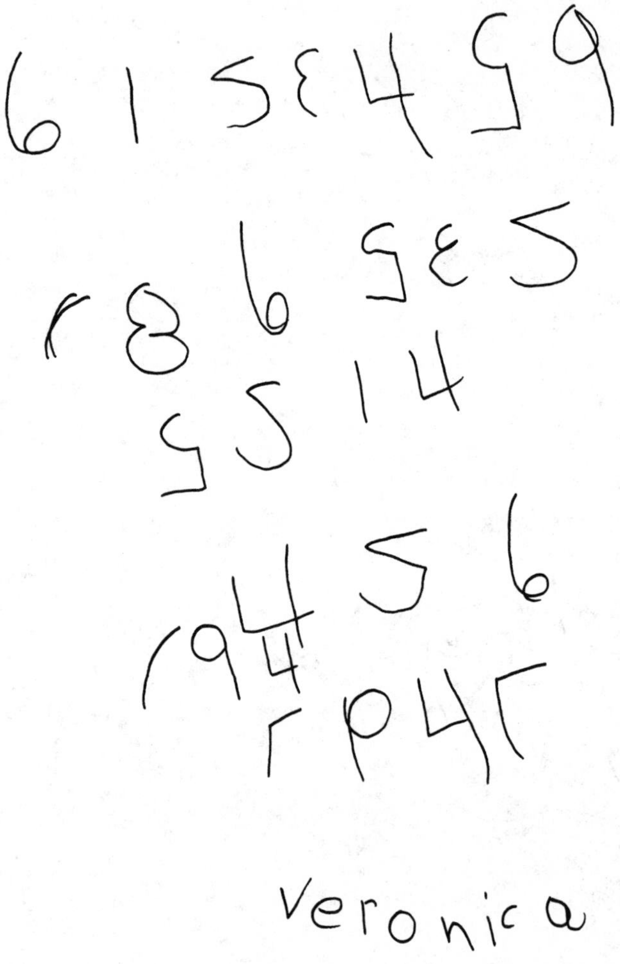

6 1 5Ƹ4 59 9

ſ 8 6 5ƸS

5 9 14

ſ94 5 6

ſ ρ 4 ſ

veronica

digits upside down: 2, 5, 6
reversals: 3, 7, 9
6 = 9

Plate 8. Veronica, C.A. 6–4.

thus her problem was not caused by poor visual perception. She had instead serious difficulties with spatial relationships, with directionality, and with visual-motor integration and written expression. She could not remember the direction of the digits when she tried to write them from recall, and had difficulty translating what she saw into writing.

Both Michelle and Veronica had serious problems with school achievement. Michelle had severe reading difficulties, whereas Veronica could read but could not write letters. Both of them required intensive training with right-left orientation, sequencing, and recall. They needed to trace and copy letters and digits until they could reproduce them automatically, and they were given lessons in tracking and spatial orientation.

Some children do not reverse digits but confuse them instead. It is not uncommon for immature kindergarten pupils to confuse 6 and 9 or 8 and 9 since these are the last digits they learn. When such a confusion occurs on the VADS Test, it is essential to find out whether the child calls a 9 consistantly "six" and calls a 6 "nine," that is, whether he recalls the correct digit but attaches the wrong label to it, or whether he uses the label "nine" and "six" interchangeably and really does not know the difference between the two digits. If the child repeats the correct digit but labels it incorrectly, then he should still get credit for his response; but if he truly confuses the two digits and cannot tell them apart, then he should not get credit for his answer.

If a youngster only knows the digits from 1 to 5 or 6, he can be given VADS Test cards that contain only the low digits. An example of this is displayed on Plate 9.

SIZE OF DIGITS

Most youngsters write the digits on the VADS Test records neither very large nor very small and they tend to make their digits uniform in size. Marked variations from this VADS Test pattern deserve attention and may reflect problems with inner control, instability, or undue anxiety and withdrawal.

Average kindergarten pupils and school beginners tend to write somewhat larger digits than older children. Plate 10 shows a good VADS Test record produced by Paula, age 5 years 8 months, a bright, well-adjusted kindergarten pupil. The digits are relatively large and even in size but, as would be expected, they are not perfect. As pointed out previously, the reversals of the 4 and 9 are quite within the normal range for kindergarten pupils. The VADS Test record of Karla, a well-functioning third-grade student, is presented on Plate 11. The digits on this record are relatively small, very neat, and well organized.

By contrast, the digits on Plate 12 are very large. They were made by Sam, age 6 years 10 months, a strong-willed, impulsive, independent, rest-

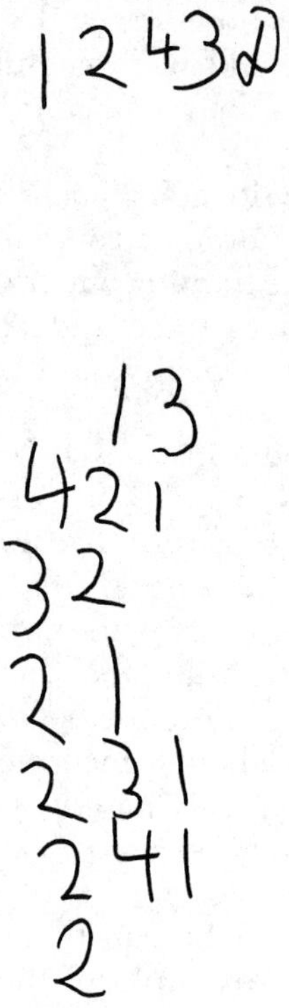

12430

13
421
32
2 1
2 31
2 41
2

digits from 1 to 4 only

Plate 9. Linda, C.A. 6–6.

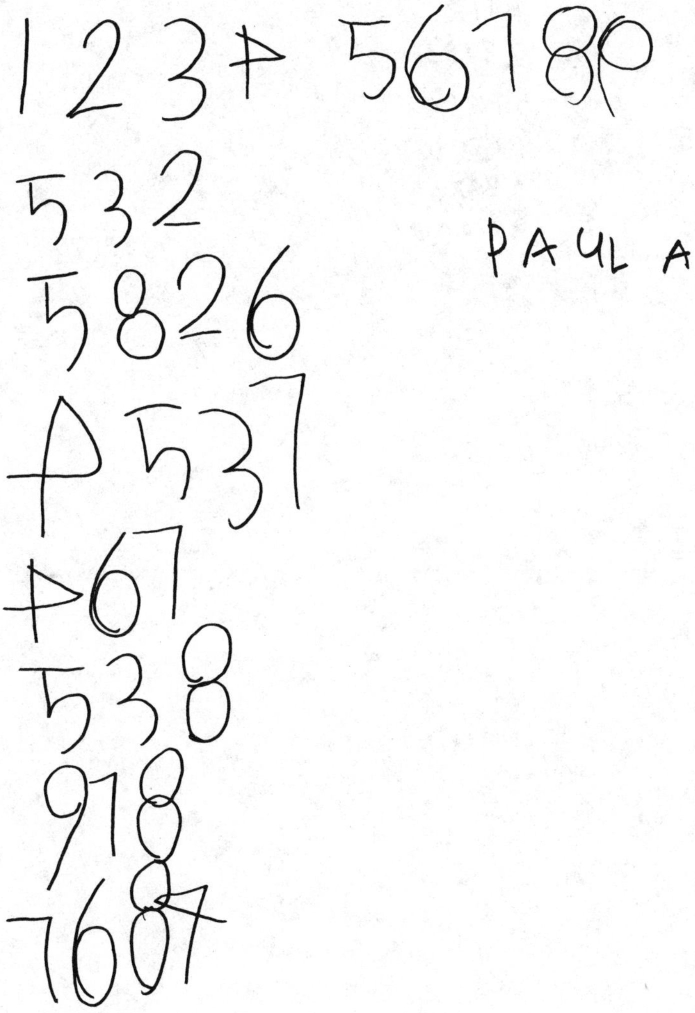

1 2 3 ♁ 5 6 7 8 ♁

5 3 2

5 8 2 6

PAUL A

♁ 5 3 7

♁ 6 7

5 3 8

9 7 8

7 6 0 7

Plate 10. Paula, C.A. 5–8.

Karla

5826   9178
96183   29763
47859   514721
47852   985216
                     389743
                     5612389

Plate 11. Karla, C.A. 8–6, third grade

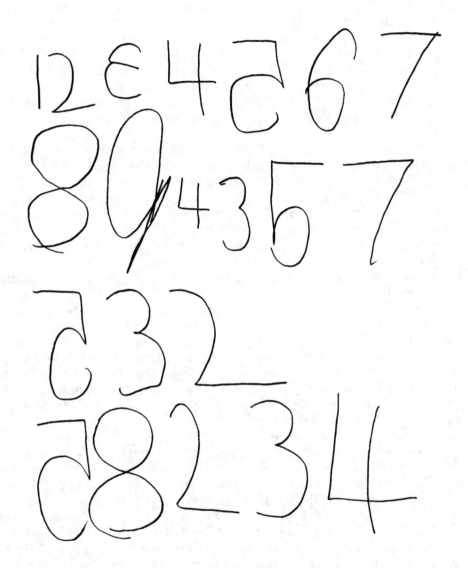

Plate 12. Sam, C.A. 6–10.

less youngster of normal mental ability. When Sam wrote the digits from 1 to 9 he increased their size as he proceded. The last digits are so large that Sam could not get them into the same row. He was only able to fit three-digit sequences of the Aural-Written Subtest on the remaining portion of the paper; Sam had to use a second sheet of paper for the Visual-Written Subtest. Once again he managed to fill the entire sheet of paper with only four-digit sequences. The largest digit on Sam's record measures no less than 4½ inches. The VADS Test record reflects vividly Sam's expansiveness and his difficulties in conforming to the rules and regulations of a regular first-grade class.

The VADS Test record on Plate 13 reveals the opposite picture. Here the digits are unusually small and decrease in size with each successive digit series. The record was produced by Gregg, age 7 years 9 months, a bright but extremely tense, insecure, and constricted second-grader, who was going through an emotional crisis following his parents' recent separation. It is interesting to note that even though Gregg was in a state of anxiety, he had no difficulty with the sequencing and recall of the digit series on the VADS Test. His VADS Test scores were all above average for his age level. His emotional problems and his anxiety were reflected in the size of his digits and not on his VADS Test scores.

Some children with emotional and behavior problems show considerable unevenness in the size of their digits on the VADS Test, just as they show unevenness in their behavior and functioning. The uneven size of the digits usually reflects impulsivity, instability, and poor inner control. Plate 14 was produced by Kim, an immature, erratic first-grader with serious behavior problems in school. He vacillated between acting-out and controlled behavior in class, just as his digits on the VADS Test record alternate between average and extremely large sizes.

Plate 15 shows a characteristic VADS Test record of a poorly controlled child with a short attention span. The VADS Test protocol was made by Yvonne, an immature 7-year-old girl who was repeating kindergarten. Yvonne was most cooperative during the administration of the VADS Test and worked very hard. She began the Aural-Written Subtest by writing very tiny digits from 1 to 9, but each succeeding digit and digit series got bigger and bigger in size. Then Yvonne paused briefly and pulled herself together. At the beginning of the Visual-Written Subtest she wrote again relatively small, well-controlled digits but her attention span was extremely short, and after a very brief time she could not muster the necessary concentration to write small, even digits. Yvonne was unable to sustain her control for any length of time. The VADS Test record was an accurate mirror of her performance in the classroom. Yvonne wanted to do her schoolwork but was too restless and distractible to stick with any task for more than a few minutes. As shown on the VADS Test, Yvonne could only handle very brief assignments and required intermittent periods of rest and change of activity. It was unrealistic to expect a child like Yvonne to finish a complete lesson in a single period.

5863
9618
38169
473769
378793,
77

9178
29763
517423
77 4825

Plate 13. Gregg, C.A. 7–9.

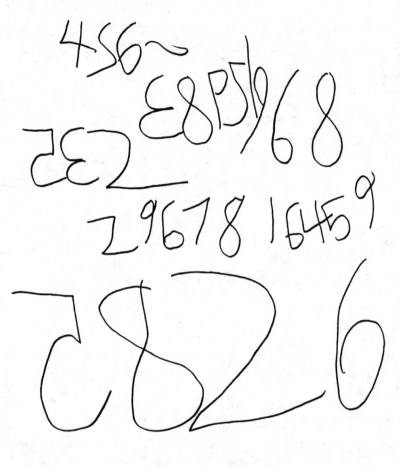

Plate 14. Kim, C.A. 6–8, first grade.

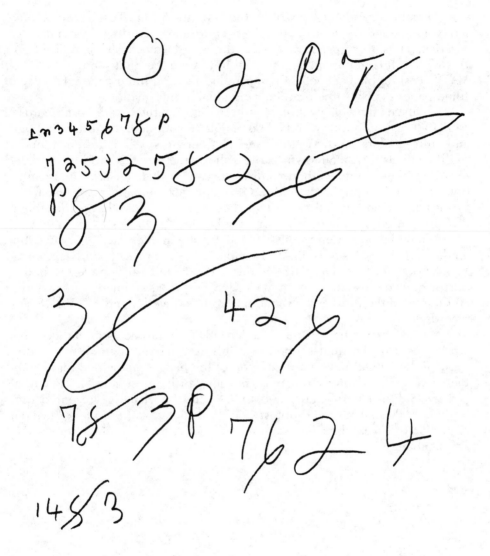

Plate 15. Yvonne, C.A. 7–0.

ORGANIZATION OF DIGITS

The organization of the written digits on the VADS Test records follows a developmental sequence and reflects children's maturity and mental organization. Thus, the organization of the digits is diagnostically significant. For this reason, it is important to have children write the digit sequences on the VADS Test on blank sheets of paper rather than on lined paper. The use of lined paper deprives the examiner of valuable information.

I analyzed the organization of written digits on the VADS Test records of 139 kindergarten pupils who had been able to complete the test, 88 second- and third-graders, and 87 fifth- and sixth-graders. All children attended public schools in a small town. Table 3 shows the way the children arranged the VADS Test digits on their records. As can be seen, changes in organization occur as the pupils get older. Only one very immature and expansive youngster spread the digits over two sheets of paper; all other youngsters in this study used one sheet of paper only for the VADS Test.

Among kindergarten pupils, 13% showed a marked lack of organization on the VADS Test records. Plates 14 and 15 are examples of poorly organized VADS Test records. Only 6% of the second- and third-graders failed to organize the digit sequences on the VADS Test in a systematic way, whereas all but one of the fifth- and six-graders produced well-organized VADS Test records.

Another immature pattern on VADS Test protocols is a horizontal arrangement of the digit sequences. Children may arrange all of the digit series in horizontal rows across the top of the page as shown on Plate 6 and Plate 16, or they may write only the auditorily presented digits (Aural-Written Subtest) horizontally and then write the visually presented digit sequences (Visual-Written Subtest) underneath each other in a vertical column. Plate 17 exhibits an example of such a mixed horizontal-vertical arrangement.

Table 3.
Organization of Digits on VADS Test Records

Pattern	Kindergarten (N 146) N	%	2nd & 3rd (N 88) N	%	5th & 6th (N 87) N	%
Use of two pages	1	1	0	0	0	0
Lack of organization	18	13	5	6	1	1
Horizontal arrangement						
Horizontal only	20	14	14	16	1	1
Horizontal & column	18	13	2	2	0	0
One column only	79	57	31	35	30	34
Two columns						
Next to each other	3	2	16	18	25	29
Underneath each other	0	0	18	20	21	24
Vertical rows	0	0	2	2	9	10

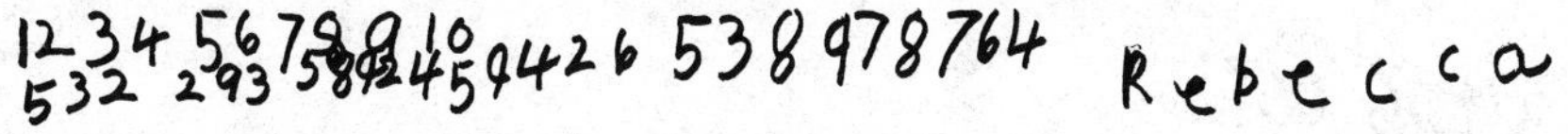

1234 5678 9 10 9426 538 978764 Rebecca
532 293 58 459

Plate 16. Rebecca, first grade.

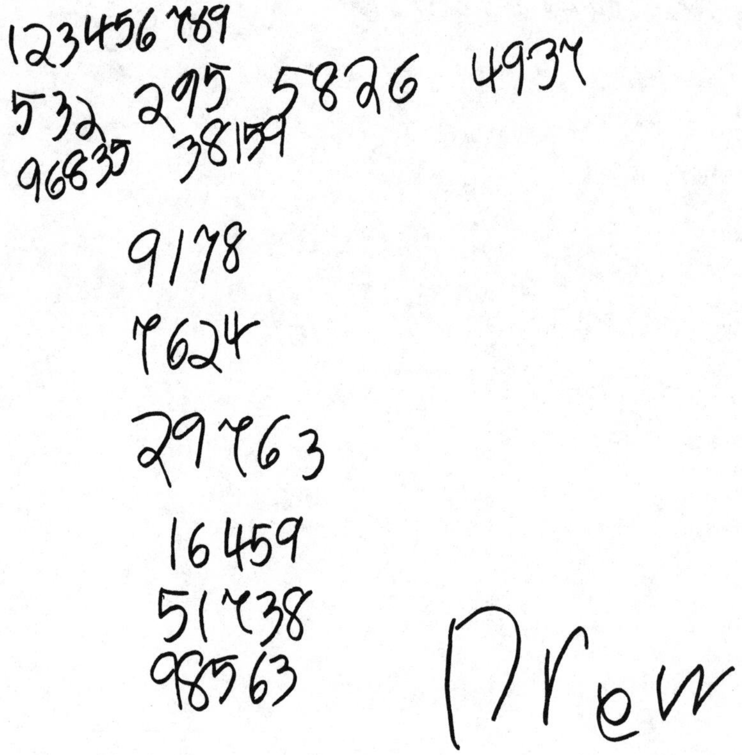

123456 789
532 295 5826 4937
96635 38159

9178

7624

29763

16459

51738
98563

Drew

Plate 17. Drew, C.A. 6–8.

More than one fourth (27%) of all kindergarten youngsters displayed either a purely horizontal or a mixed horizontal-vertical organization of the digit sequences on their VADS Test records; 16% of the second- and third-graders used horizontal arrangements, but hardly any of them revealed a mixed horizontal-vertical organization on their VADS Test protocols. They seem to use either only a horizontal or only a vertical arrangement. It is apparently most unusual to find a VADS Test record with a horizontal arrangement of digit series among fifth- and sixth-graders. When it does occur it reflects usually marked immaturity.

The most commonly shown pattern on VADS Test records is the arrangement of digit sequences in a vertical column, either in single columns or in double columns. Single columns are usually placed on the left-hand side of the paper, or less often, down the middle of the page. A single column arrangement was used by more than half (57%) of all kindergarten pupils, and by roughly one-third of the two groups of older pupils. A typical record of this kind was shown on Plate 10.

The arrangement of digit sequences into two columns indicates mental maturity and good organization. Only 2% of the kindergarten youngsters employed this form of digit arrangement, whereas, 38% of the second- and third-graders, and 53% of the fifth- and sixth-graders wrote the digit series in two distinct columns, either placed next to each other as shown on Plate 11, or beneath each other as shown on Plate 13.

A small number of pupils wrote the auditorily presented digits of a series (Aural-Written Subtest) in vertical rows, like the scores on a scoring sheet or like the digits of an addition problem. When the digit sequences were then presented visually (Visual-Written Subtest), some of the youngsters switched from a vertical row arrangement of the digits to a column organization. Plates 18 and 19 illustrate vertical rows and a vertical row and column arrangement on VADS Test records. Either type of organization seems to occur primarily among older children.

Thus, we can see on Table 3 that there is a developmental sequence in the organization of digit series on VADS Test records. Very young children are not yet able to write digits; when they first begin to write digits they do so without any meaningful organization. As the youngsters mature they use a horizontal arrangement of the digit series; this changes either gradually or abruptly into a column organization, that is, the digit series are placed underneath each other in a column. More mature pupils use two columns, one for the Aural-Written and one for the Visual-Written digit sequences. The two columns can be placed next to each other or beneath each other. A small group of individualistic youngsters place the single digits within a given sequence under each other in vertical rows. This type of arrangement occurs mainly among older children.

The majority of elementary school children seem to arrange the digit series in one or two columns on the VADS Test records. A lack of organization or a horizontal arrangement of digits reflects immaturity. When these types of arrangements are found on the VADS Test records of older pupils, they indicate a developmental lag or poor mental organization.

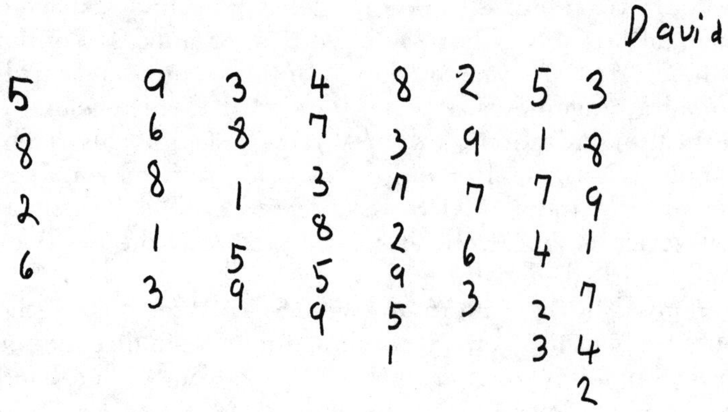

David

5	9	3	4	8	2	5	3
8	6	8	7	3	9	1	8
2	8	1	3	7	7	7	9
6	1	5	8	2	6	4	1
	3	9	5	9	3	2	7
			9	5		3	4
				1			2

Plate 18. David, sixth grade.

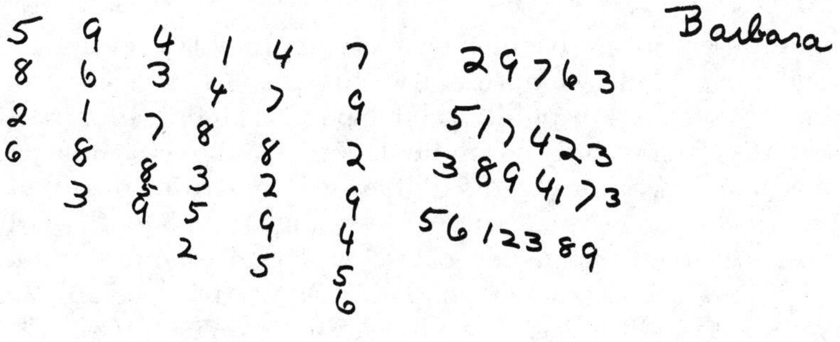

Barbara

```
5   9   4   1   4   7    2 9 7 6 3
8   6   3   4   7   9    5 1 7 4 2 3
2   1   7   8   7   2    3 8 9 4 7 3
6   8   8   3   8   9    5 6 1 2 3 8 9
    3   9   3   2   4
            5   9   4
            2   5   5
                    6
```

Plate 19. Barbara, sixth grade.

CORRECTIONS ON THE VADS TEST RECORDS

Many children are aware of their errors when they are recalling digit sequences, and some of the youngsters try spontaneously to correct them. Approximately 7% of the 419 public school pupils, kindergarten to sixth grade, whose VADS Test records I examined, erased and rewrote one or two digits, whereas another 7% corrected a digit or two by writing over them. A child rarely corrected more than one or two digits, and most of these corrections were relatively neatly executed. A typical example of such a corrected VADS Test record is shown on Plate 20. It was produced by Victor, age 12 years 4 months. On the Visual-Written Subtest, Victor wrote 29363, then he corrected the first 3 by writing a 7 over it. On the following digit sequence Victor wrote a 2 over the second 5. In both cases he corrected errors he had made.

Kindergarten pupils and first-graders sometimes erase a digit that had been reversed. In such instances, the correction merely involves the writing of the digit but not a change of the digit. Older children tend to change one digit into another one when they erase or write over digits. All such deliberate, and usually successful, corrections on the VADS Test can be regarded as positive signs; they tend to reflect good inner control and intelligence on the part of the youngsters involved. These kinds of corrections are quite different from the impulsive scribbling over or crossing out of digits that are occasionally found on the VADS Test records of aggressive, acting-out youngsters, or on the protocols of children with low frustration tolerance and poor inner control.

Examples of such scribbled over and crossed out digit sequences are shown on Plate 4 and Plate 21. It is extremely rare to find a scribbled over VADS Test record among normal, well-functioning public school pupils. The VADS Test record on Plate 21 was produced by Gary, age 12 years 11 months. He was an impulsive, hypersensitive, insecure youngster with serious behavior and learning problems. His attention span was very short and his frustration tolerance was minimal. Gary was quite verbal and repeated the five-, six-, and seven-digit sequences on the Aural-Oral and Visual-Oral VADS Subtests without effort, but aural-written integration was hard for him. He wrote the four- and five-digit series on the Aural-Written Subtest without error; on the six-digit series Gary had difficulty with the sequencing. He was aware of his errors and impulsively crossed out the incorrect responses and tried to rewrite them no less than seven times. In the meantime he had forgotten most of the digits and became extremely frustrated. He jumped up and was ready to quit.

With a bit of encouragement and persuasion on my part, Gary was willing to try the Visual-Written Subtest. He reproduced all of the digit-sequences with only one minor error that he corrected by writing over the incorrect digit.

Gary's performance on the VADS Test was typical of his classroom behavior. He worked very fast and did not analyze problems or plan his answers. He just forged ahead impulsively and crossed out or even destroyed his work when he thought he was failing or did not know an answer.

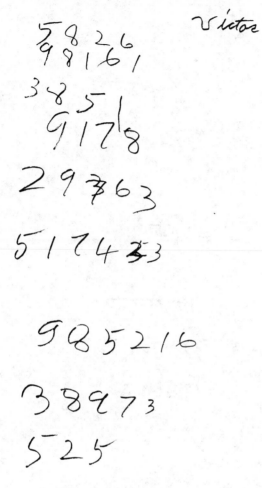

Plate 20. Victor, C.A. 12–4.

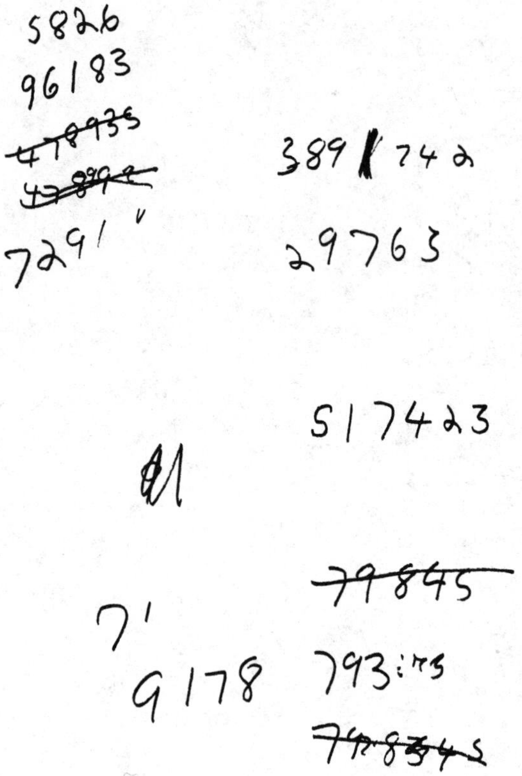

5826

96183

~~78935~~

~~899~~

729¹ ''

389 ╱ 74 2

29763

517423

01

79845

7¹

9178   793:73

~~78345~~

Plate 21. Gary, C.A. 12–11.

NUMBERING AND LINES ON VADS TEST RECORDS

A blank sheet of paper presents a challenge for many youngsters when writing the VADS Test digits. Bright and well-controlled children tend to arrange the digits spontaneously into columns and thus structure the field to suit their needs. But disorganized and impulsive pupils are often uncomfortable with blank sheets of paper, and need external limits and structure as guidelines when writing digit series. They frequently attempt to provide structure for themselves when it has not been provided by the examiner. On VADS Test records, such structure may take the form of numbering the digit sequences or of underlining or enclosing the digit series with lines.

Plate 22 shows the highly structured VADS Test record of Donna, age 11 years 4 months. She numbered each of the digit series and lined them up along the outer edge of the paper. She also drew a line under the last Aural-Written sequence in order to separate it from the Visual-Written digit series. Donna obtained a perfect score on the VADS Test, and she was an outstanding sixth-grade pupil. She was a deliberate, methodical worker who carefully planned and structured her schoolwork, but she could not be rushed. When pressured to work fast she became disorganized.

Some youngsters underline digit series on the VADS Test records, or they may draw an enclosure or box around some or all of the digit sequences. Such lines and enclosures are quite similar in nature to the boxes found on Bender Gestalt Test protocols and can be interpreted in the same way (Koppitz, 1975a, p. 86). Lines and enclosures occurred only on 2% of the 419 VADS Test records of normal public school pupils, kindergarten to sixth grade, that I examined.

When children draw lines or enclosures on the VADS Test records, they are showing us that they are impulsive and need limits, and that they feel uncomfortable with wide open, unstructured situations or spaces. The majority of youngsters with behavior and learning problems are impulsive and poorly controlled. It comes, therefore, as no surprise that they also produce much more often lines and enclosures on the VADS Test records then average public school pupils. The VADS Test records shown on Plates 23, 24, 25, and 26 were all made by educationally handicapped pupils who were attending special education classes.

The VADS Test record on Plate 23 was made by Bob, age 9 years 7 months; he was a neurologically impaired, impulsive, disorganized youngster with very poor fine-motor coordination. Writing was difficult for Bob, as can be readily seen on his VADS Test record. Bob held his pencil awkwardly and wrote very slowly and with effort. He carefully underlined each digit sequence to help him organize his work. Without such rigid structure he was unable to focus and to follow through on his work. But even with this aid his concentration was poor and his attention span was short.

Plate 24 shows Karl's VADS Test record. Karl was a hypertalkative, restless, impulsive 11-year-old boy, of average mental ability, with serious learning problems. When taking the VADS Test, he was eager to please and put forth much effort. His VADS Test protocol is unusual in that he drew a

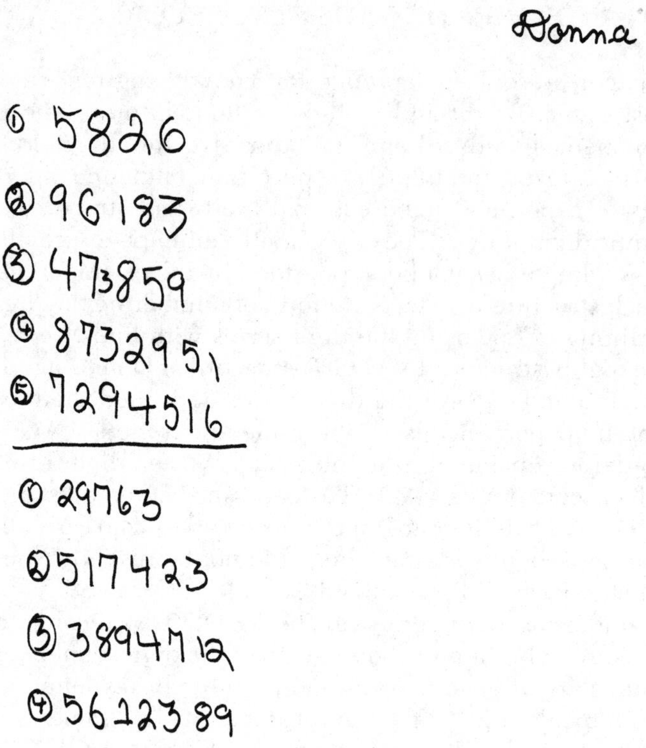

Donna

① 5826

② 96183

③ 473859

④ 8732951

⑤ 7294516

_____

① 29763

② 517423

③ 3894712

④ 5612389

Plate 22. Donna, C.A. 11–4.

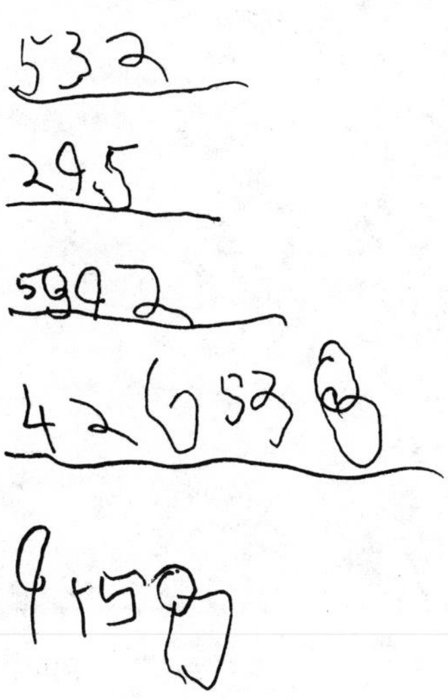

532

295

5942

426538

9159

Plate 23. Bob, C.A. 9-7.

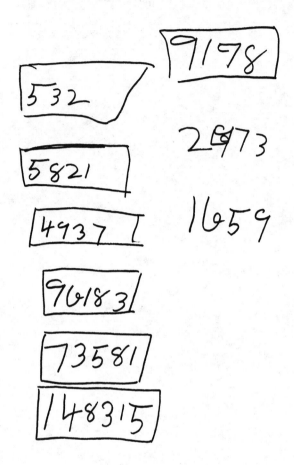

Plate 24. Karl, C.A. 11–8.

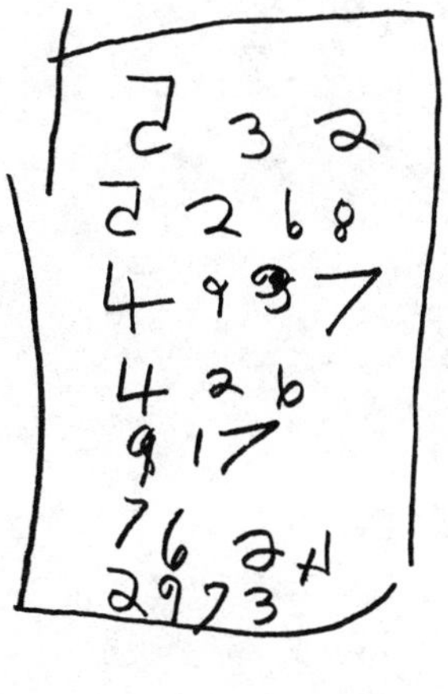

Plate 25. Sandra, C.A. 7–6.

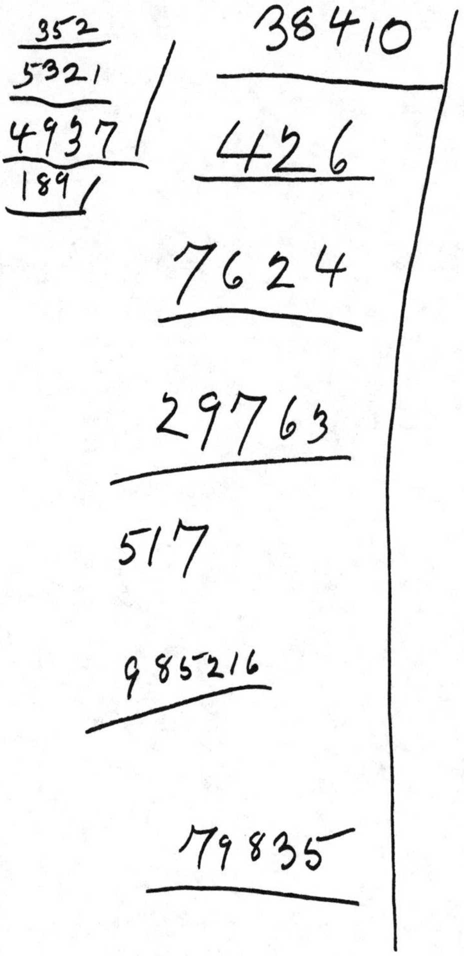

352
5321
4937
189

38410

426

7624

29763

517

985216

79835

Plate 26. Cynthia, C.A. 9–3.

box around each digit sequence after he had completed it. The VADS Test record reflects Karl's behavior in the classroom. Karl could only complete assignments that were brief, quite explicit, and highly structured; he got distracted and disorganized when he was given long or unstructured work. Karl always had to finish one problem and "wrap it up" before he could begin the next one, just as he placed his completed answers on the VADS Test in a box before he proceeded to the next one.

Sandra, age 7 years 6 months, was even more impulsive than Karl, but she lacked his intelligence. She was an immature, emotionally deprived child of borderline mental ability. Sandra had a long history of aggressive, acting-out behavior. In the small, highly structured special class, Sandra did reasonably well as long as she had a supportive but firm teacher. When she was moved to a less structured teacher, Sandra regressed to her former unsocialized, disruptive behavior. Plate 25 shows her VADS Test record. The record dramatically reveals Sandra's need for outer control and limits; she enclosed all of her digit sequences with a line as though they might fall apart if no limits were placed around them, just as she herself lost control over her impulses when no outer controls were provided.

Cynthia, age 9 years 3 months, displayed both underlining and enclosures of the digit series on her VADS Test record, as shown on Plate 26. Cynthia was another impulsive, acting-out child with severe language and learning problems. She too required a great deal of external structure and control to keep her from fighting with peers and to get her to complete her assignments. On the VADS Test, Cynthia showed that she could structure and organize her work when she was given individual encouragement and support.

Bob, Karl, Sandra, and Cynthia, were all extremely impulsive and had weak inner control and organization. They all needed and wanted outer controls to guide them and to set limits for them. The lines and enclosures they drew on their VADS Test records (Plates 23, 24, 25, and 26) reflect this need graphically.

ANALYSIS OF VADS TEST RECORDS: SUMMARY

VADS Test records can be analyzed in several different ways so as to yield valuable diagnostic information. The formation, size, and arrangement of digits on the VADS Test records follow a developmental sequence. Marked deviations in either direction from the normal developmental sequence can reflect either good maturation and mental ability, especially in young children, or significant immaturity, a developmental lag, or specific problems that are often associated with learning problems.

Digit reversals are common among kindergarten pupils but not among older children. Digit reversals and inversions, and the writing of digit sequences from right to left, may reflect difficulties with directionality and spatial relationships. Unusually *large digits* are often associated with immaturity, expansiveness, and poor inner control; *very small* digits show tense-ness, insecurity, anxiety, withdrawal, and constriction. *Uneven digits* are most often produced by unstable, erratic, and impulsive children, whereas an *increasing size* of digits is typical for youngsters with a short attention span, low frustration tolerance, and poor inner control. A *decrease in digit size* indicates withdrawal. Very young children show little *organization of digit series* on the VADS Test records; as pupils mature they place the digit sequences in horizontal rows, then in horizontal-vertical arrangements, and finally, in one or two columns or in vertical rows of single digits. The type of digit arrangement shown on a VADS Test record reveals the pupil's level of mental maturity and organization.

Spontaneous corrections or digit changes on VADS Test records suggest good control and intelligence, whereas scribbling over or crossing out of digits suggest poor inner control, impulsivity, acting-out behavior, and aggressiveness. Children who are trying to control their impulsivity often number the digit sequences or draw lines or boxes around them, thereby showing their need for structure, outer limits, and control.

Chapter 6

Scoring of the VADS Test

The scoring of the VADS Test is very simple. The score for a given VADS Subtest equals the longest digit sequence that a child is able to recall without errors. Thus, if a pupil repeats correctly the first four-digit sequence on the Aural-Oral Subtest, then misses the first five-digit series but gets the second five-digit sequence, and thereafter fails both of the six-digit sequences, then his score for this Subtest would be 5. If the child passes either the first or second five-digit sequence and six-digit sequence on the Visual-Oral Subtest, only to miss both trials on the seven-digit series, then his score on the Visual-Oral Subtest would be 6, and so on. The highest Subtest score a youngster can obtain on any of the four Subtests is 7, since the longest digit sequence presented contains seven digits.

The VADS Test yields three different types of test scores: the scores for the four Subtests, the six scores for the various combinations of the Subtest scores, and the Total VADS Test score. In all, 11 different VADS Test measures can be obtained from a single VADS Test performance:

VADS Subtests
  1. Aural-Oral or A-O
  2. Visual-Oral or V-O
  3. Aural-Written or A-W
  4. Visual-Written or V-W
VADS Combination Scores
  5. Aural Input or A I (A-O & A-W)
  6. Visual Input or V I (V-O & V-W)
  7. Oral Expression or O E (A-O & V-O)
  8. Written Expression or W E (A-W & V-W)
  9. Intrasensory Integration or Intra (A-O & V-W)
 10. Intersensory Integration or Inter (V-O & A-W)
 11. *Total VADS Test Score* or. Total (A-O & V-O & A-W & V-W)

The score range of the four VADS Subtests extends from 0 to 7. The six VADS Combination measures have a score range from 0 to 14, which allows for a good discrimination between children's test performances. This is even more true for the Total VADS Test score, which extends theoretically from 0 to 28. However, if a child is unable to reproduce a single digit on any of the VADS Subtests, then the test is obviously not appropriate for the youngster.

Each of the four VADS Subtests measures a somewhat different aspect of perceptual-motor integration, sequencing, and recall. The Combined and Total VADS Test scores are, of course, interrelated since they are derived from the four Subtests. Carr (1974) explored the degree of interrelatedness of ten of the eleven VADS Test measures (the Intrasensory Integration score was not included in the study) by correlating the VADS Test scores of 26 fourth-grade pupils. Table 4 shows the results.

Table 4.
Correlations Between VADS Test Scores[1]

VADS	A–O	V–O	A–W	V–W	A I	V I	O E	W E	Inter	Total
A–O		.29	.61**	.27	.88**	.33	.86**	.56**	.52**	.77**
V–O			.33	.41*	.34	.78**	.73**	.46*	.68**	.65**
A–W				.25	.91**	.33	.60**	.82**	.73**	.79**
V–W					.29	.89**	.41*	.77**	.50**	.67**
A I						.37	.81**	.78**	.70**	.87**
V I							.65**	.76**	.68**	.78**
O E								.65**	.73**	.89**
W E									.78**	.92**
Inter										.83**

[1]The data are here reproduced with permission of Margaret Carr, Fort Worth, Texas (1974).
*Correlation significant at the .05 level.
**Correlation significant at the .01 level.

Six of the VADS Test measures (A-O, V-O, A-W, V-W, A I, V I) were significantly related ($p \leqslant .01$) to the Total VADS Test and to the Oral Expression, Written Expression, and Intersensory Integration scores. The Oral Expression, Written Expression, Intersensory Integration, and Total VADS Test scores all include both aural and visual presentation of digits, they were also all closely interrelated. The degree to which the VADS Test measures were interrelated seemed to depend to a large extent on the mode in which the digit sequences were presented. When the mode of input differed (aural versus visual), then the correlation between the VADS Test measures was low. The correlations between the three VADS Test measures with only auditory presentation of digit-series (A-O, A-W, A I) and the three measures with only visual input (V-O, V-W, V I) were positive but low; none of them was statistically significant.

A youngster's VADS Test scores can be compared to those of other children of his age or grade level, and can also be compared to each other. Experience has shown that the various VADS Test score patterns have considerable diagnostic value.

The four VADS Subtests measure children's ability for processing, integration, sequencing, and recall. Each of these Subtests is quite distinct, and a child may do well or poorly in any one of them and not in the others. It makes a great deal of difference whether a pupil has difficulty with only one of the four VADS Subtests or with all four of them. If a pupil gets a low score only on the Visual-Oral Subtest, for instance, whereas his Aural-Oral, Aural-Written, and Visual-Written Subtest scores are average, then he may have a specific disability in visual-oral integration and recall. If, on the other hand, all four VADS Subtest scores are low, then the youngster may be immature and may have problems with intersensory integration and memory for symbols, in general. In that case, the low VADS Test scores may reflect an overall limitation in the child's mental processing rather than a specific disability.

Of particular significance are the comparisons between the various VADS Test Combination scores. For example, if a pupil has a high score on Aural Input (A-O & A-W) and a low score on Visual Input (V-O & V-W) then one can assume that the youngster has difficulty with the processing and recall of visually presented symbols and does not have problems in the area of expression or integration. The Aural Input and Visual Input scores each include one Subtest with oral expression and one with written expression, and one Subtest with intrasensory integration and one with intersensory integration, therefore the modes of expression and integration are controlled on both the Aural and Visual Input scores.

In a case where a youngster has a markedly higher Oral Expression score (A-O & V-O) than a Written Expression score (A-W & V-W), the child has most likely difficulty getting things down on paper from memory. These differences in the test scores cannot be the result of the mode of presenting the digits or of the mode of integration, since both of these have been controlled. The Oral Expression and the Written Expression scores each include one Subtest with aural and one with visual input, and one Subtest with intrasensory and one with intersensory integration.

And finally, one can compare pupils' Intrasensory Integration scores (A-O & V-W) with their Intersensory Integration scores (V-O & A-W). The Intrasensory Integration score includes the two VADS Subtests that operate within the same sense modality for both input and output, that is, Aural-Oral operates within the auditory mode and Visual-Written operates in the visual mode. By contrast, the Intersensory Integration scores are based on the two VADS Subtests that involve the integration of two different sense modalities, that is, the integration of the visual and the auditory modes. If a youngster has a low score on Intrasensory Integration and a high score on Intersensory Integration, then his problems are most likely the result of specific difficulties with intrasensory integration and not of problems with the modes of input or expression, as these were controlled. The Intrasensory Integration and Intersensory Integration scores each include one VADS Subtest with aural and one with visual presentation, and one Subtest with oral and one with written expression.

The Total VADS Test score measures the entire process of perceptual-motor integration, sequencing, and recall. It reflects the youngsters' overall functioning in these areas. Perceptual-motor integration, sequencing, and recall of symbols are closely related to school learning and to achievement. The various VADS Subtest and Combination scores are especially useful in diagnosing specific areas of strength and weakness in a child and in discovering his preferred mode of perception and expression. The 11 VADS Test measures can be very helpful, as part of a test battery, when prescribing and developing meaningful educational programs for youngsters with specific learning difficulties.

RELIABILITY OF VADS TEST

The reliability of the VADS Test was determined by the test-retest method. The subjects for this study were two groups of youngsters with learning and behavior problems to whom I had given the VADS Test twice. The interval between the first and second administration of the VADS Test ranged from 1 day to 15 weeks; the mean interval for both groups was 6½ weeks. The first group of pupils included 35 6- to 10-year-olds, whereas the second group was made up of 27 11- and 12-year-old students. For each of the groups, Pearson product moment coefficients were computed between the two sets of VADS Test scores.

Table 5 shows the results for the two groups of subjects. All 11 correlations for the 6- to 10- and the 11- and 12-year-old children were statistically significant at the .001 level. Thus, it appears that the VADS Test scores are quite reliable over a 3- to 4-month period for elementary school youngsters with learning and behavior problems. Since children with behavior and learning difficulties tend to be more unstable than well-functioning pupils, it is hypothesized that the VADS Test is also reliable for average schoolchildren.

Table 5.
Test-Retest on the VADS Test Correlations

VADS	CA 6 to 10 (N 35)	CA 11 and 12 (N 27)
Aural-Oral	.84	.85
Visual-Oral	.74	.84
Aural-Written	.78	.72
Visual-Written	.77	.80
Aural Input	.85	.87
Visual Input	.90	.88
Oral Expression	.84	.79
Written Expression	.82	.80
Intrasensory Integration	.87	.87
Intersensory Integration	.85	.86
Total VADS	.92	.90

Chapter 7

VADS Test Normative Data

NORMATIVE SAMPLE

The VADS Test normative data were derived from 810 normal public school pupils, kindergarten through sixth grade. The youngsters ranged in age from 5 years 6 months to 12 years 11 months. No children with serious physical or mental handicaps were included in the normative sample. The pupils represent a socioeconomic cross section and came from upper-middle, middle-, lower-middle class, and deprived home backgrounds. Of the children tested 16% came from large cities, 59% lived in small or medium-sized cities, 20% had homes in suburban communities, and the remaining 6% came from rural areas or villages. The majority of youngsters (69%) lived in the Northeast (New York State), but the Midwest (Ohio) and the West (California) also each contributed 12% to the normative sample; an additional 6% lived in the South (Virginia and Texas).

The 810 pupils were about evenly divided among boys and girls. Table 6 shows the sex distribution and the ethnic grouping for each age level, $5\frac{1}{2}$ to 12 years. Of the children 81% were white, 13% were black, 6% were Hispanic, and less than 1% was Oriental. The VADS Test was administered individually to all children by qualified psychologists.

Only one brief study has thus far investigated group differences on the VADS Test. Millavec (1971) administered the VADS Test to 15 pairs of matched black and white youngsters age $4\frac{1}{2}$ to $7\frac{1}{2}$. Millavec reported that the black children performed significantly better on the Aural-Oral Subtest than the white children ($p < .05$). Since most of the youngsters were still too immature to complete the entire VADS Test, no other statistical analysis was possible.

Bridgeman and Buttram (1975) compared the Digit Span Test performance of 100 white and 100 black fourth- and fifth-grade pupils in rural Virginia. They found no significant differences between the two groups on the recall of three- to nine-digit series. A comparison of VADS Test records of different socio-cultural groups will have to wait for future research.

SEX DIFFERENCE ON THE VADS TEST

In an earlier study (Koppitz, 1970), I compared the VADS Test scores of 50 pairs of boys and girls, matched for age and IQ scores. The youngsters ranged in age from $6\frac{1}{2}$ to 11 years and attended first to fifth grade. Statistical analysis failed to show any significant differences between the VADS Subtests and the Total VADS Test score of the boys and girls.

Table 6.

Sex Distribution and Ethnic Grouping of Normative Sample

Age	Boys N	Girls N	Total N	White N	White %	Black N	Black %	Hispanic N	Hispanic %	Oriental N	Oriental %
5–6/5–11	37	39	76	61	80	10	13	3	4	2	3
6–0/6–5	49	52	101	85	84	13	13	3	3	0	0
6–6/6–11	35	40	75	61	81	9	12	4	5	1	1
7–0/7–5	42	38	80	66	82	10	13	4	5	0	0
7–6/7–11	47	50	97	78	80	12	12	7	7	0	0
8–0/8–11	47	47	94	79	84	11	12	4	4	0	0
9–0/9–11	41	39	80	65	82	9	11	5	6	1	1
10–0/10–11	41	41	82	68	83	10	12	4	5	0	0
11–0/11–11	40	40	80	57	71	13	16	9	11	1	1
12–0/12–11	23	22	45	35	78	5	11	5	11	0	0
Total	402	408	810	655	81	102	13	48	6	5	6

Most recently, I compared the VADS Test performance of 40 boys and 40 girls who were completing kindergarten. Once again, the results showed no statistically significant differences between the VADS Test scores of the two groups. Because of these findings, only one set of VADS Test norms for both boys and girls is presented.

VADS TEST NORMS

The VADS Test normative data are presented in five different ways so that a given youngster's VADS Test scores can be compared to the VADS Test scores of other children of the same age level and the same grade level, and to children whose VADS Test performance resembles his own. The five sets of VADS Test normative data include:

1. Means and Standard Deviations by age level for children age 5½ to 12.
2. Percentile scores by age level for children age 5½ to 12.
3. Age equivalents for Total VADS Test scores.
4. Means and Standard Deviations by grade level, K to sixth grade.
5. Percentile scores by grade level, K to sixth grade.

MEANS AND STANDARD DEVIATIONS BY AGE LEVEL

The means and standard deviations for the eleven VADS Test measures were computed for each age level, 5½ to 12 years. Between age 5½ and age 7, a great deal of maturation and learning takes place in perceptual-motor integration and in reading and writing; hence there is a marked increase in the VADS Test scores during this age span. Thereafter, the increment in VADS Test scores is more gradual. Therefore, the VADS Test norms are given in 6-month intervals for the younger children and in 12-month intervals for pupils age 7 and older. Table 7 shows the VADS Test means and standard deviations for each age level, as well as plus-minus one standard deviation from the mean, or the normal range of VADS Test scores.

The graph on Figure 1 depicts the mean scores of the four VADS Subtests for the normative sample. The graph demonstrates clearly that the VADS Test scores of schoolchildren are related to their age level; that is, the scores improve steadily between the age of 5½ and 12. These findings are consistent with the results of other studies with memory span tests. There is a consensus that children's memory span increases with age (Alwitt, 1963; Birch and Belmont, 1965 b; Daehler et al., 1969; Flavell et al., 1966; Kahn and Birch, 1968; London and Robinson, 1968; Murray and Roberts, 1968; Senf 1969; Wachs, 1969). Most likely, both maturation and learning contribute to this improvement. The increase in VADS Test Scores seems to depend to a large extent on a gradual improvement in children's recall strategies. Older children tend to organize, chunk, and rehearse digits more often and more effectively than younger children; these procedures facilitate the recall of digit sequences.

Table 7.
VADS Test Mean Scores and Standard Deviations for Age 5½ to 12

VADS	CA 5-6/5-11 (N 76)			CA 6-0/6-5 (N 101)			CA 6-6/6-11 (N 75)		
	Mean	S.D.	±1 S.D.	Mean	S.D.	±1 S.D.	Mean	S.D.	±1 S.D.
A-O	3.97	.71	3.3-4.7	4.23	.89	3.3-5.1	4.56	.74	3.8-5.3
V-O	3.67	1.29	2.4-5.0	4.12	1.10	3.0-5.2	4.81	.70	4.1-5.5
A-W	2.76	1.19	1.6-4.0	3.12	1.13	2.0-4.3	4.09	1.00	3.0-5.0
V-W	3.04	1.33	1.7-4.4	3.50	1.28	2.2-4.8	4.53	.79	3.7-5.3
A I	6.74	1.67	5.0-8.4	7.35	1.74	5.6-9.1	8.66	1.45	7.2-10.1
V I	6.72	2.41	4.3-9.1	7.57	2.18	5.4-9.8	9.35	1.30	8.1-10.7
O E	7.65	1.86	5.8-9.5	8.31	1.80	6.5-10.11	9.39	1.31	8.1-10.7
W E	5.80	2.40	3.4-8.2	6.61	2.25	4.4-8.9	8.63	1.55	7.1-10.2
Intra	7.01	1.79	5.2-8.8	7.72	1.85	5.9-9.6	9.11	1.26	7.9-10.4
Inter	6.45	2.28	4.2-8.7	7.20	2.05	5.2-9.3	8.91	1.44	7.5-10.4
Total	13.46	3.91	9.6-17.5	14.92	3.67	11.3-18.6	18.03	2.61	15.4-20.6

VADS	CA 7-0/7-11 (N 177)			CA 8-0/8-11 (N 94)			CA 9-0/9-11 (N 80)		
	Mean	S.D.	±1 S.D.	Mean	S.D.	±1 S.D.	Mean	S.D.	±1 S.D.
A-O	5.12	.95	4.2-6.1	5.22	.89	4.3-6.1	5.43	.99	4.4-6.4
V-O	5.31	1.10	4.2-6.4	5.58	.95	4.6-6.5	5.91	1.09	4.8-7.0
A-W	4.79	.97	3.8-5.8	4.78	.94	3.8-5.7	5.19	1.01	4.2-6.2
V-W	5.10	1.24	3.9-6.3	5.56	1.02	4.5-6.6	5.89	1.10	4.8-7.0
A I	9.91	1.67	8.2-11.6	10.00	1.60	8.4-11.6	10.61	1.82	8.8-12.4
V I	10.42	2.04	8.4-12.5	11.14	1.73	9.4-12.9	11.80	1.96	9.8-13.8
O E	10.42	1.72	8.7-12.1	10.80	1.49	9.3-12.3	11.34	1.76	9.6-13.1
W E	9.90	1.84	8.1-11.7	10.34	1.64	8.7-12.0	11.08	1.85	9.2-12.9
Intra	10.24	1.72	8.5-12.0	10.78	1.61	9.2-12.4	11.31	1.75	9.6-13.1
Inter	10.09	1.80	8.3-11.9	10.35	1.59	8.8-10.4	11.10	1.78	9.3-12.9
Total	20.32	3.25	17.1-23.6	21.14	2.88	18.3-24.0	22.41	3.32	19.1-25.7

Table 7. (continued)

VADS Test Mean Scores and Standard Deviations for Age 5½ to 12

VADS	CA 10-0/10-11 (N 82)			CA 11-0/11-11 (N 80)			CA 12-0/12-11 (N 45)		
	Mean	S.D.	±1 S.D.	Mean	S.D.	±1 S.D.	Mean	S.D.	±1 S.D.
A-O	5.89	.92	5.0-6.8	5.95	.83	5.1-6.8	6.27	.86	5.4-7.1
V-O	6.34	.82	5.5-7.0	6.54	.73	5.8-7.0	6.62	.65	6.0-7.3
A-W	5.48	1.06	4.4-6.5	5.74	1.04	4.7-6.8	6.09	.95	5.1-7.0
V-W	6.43	.72	5.7-7.0	6.56	.69	5.9-7.0	6.69	.63	6.0-7.3
A I	11.35	1.75	9.6-13.1	11.69	1.63	10.1-13.3	12.36	1.51	10.9-13.9
V I	12.77	1.32	11.5-14.0	13.10	1.19	11.9-14.0	13.31	1.04	12.3-14.4
O E	12.23	1.39	10.8-13.6	12.49	1.26	11.2-13.8	12.89	1.19	11.7-14.1
W E	11.90	1.55	10.4-13.5	12.30	1.47	10.8-13.8	12.78	1.30	11.5-14.1
Intra	12.32	1.35	11.0-13.7	12.51	1.18	11.3-13.7	12.96	1.26	11.7-14.1
Inter	11.82	1.60	10.2-13.4	12.28	1.52	10.8-13.8	12.71	1.18	11.5-13.9
Total	24.13	2.69	21.4-26.8	24.79	2.45	22.3-27.2	25.67	2.12	23.6-27.8

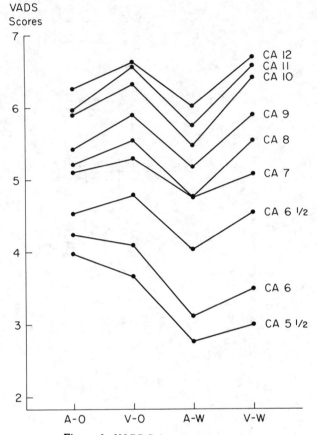

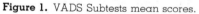

Figure 1. VADS Subtests mean scores.

The graph on Figure 1 also shows the characteristic shape of the VADS Subtest score distribution for all age levels from age 6½ to age 12, or for first- to sixth-graders. From age 6½ on, the mode of presentation, aural versus visual, has a greater effect on the VADS Test scores than the mode of expression. The two VADS Subtests with visual input, the Visual-Oral and Visual-Written Subtests, show consistently higher scores than the two VADS Subtests with aural input, the Aural-Oral and Aural-Written Subtests.

Kindergarten pupils and very immature youngsters reveal a slightly different VADS Test score pattern. The 5½- and 6-year-old children tend to do best on the Aural-Oral Subtest and only slightly less well on the Visual-Oral Subtest. Both of these scores are much better than the Aural-Written and Visual-Written Subtest scores. Very young children are more successful when they can say the digit sequences instead of having to write them. This is not surprising since many kindergarten youngsters still have difficulty with the writing of digits. It follows, therefore, that for the 5½- and 6-year-olds, the mode of expression, oral versus written, influences the VADS Test scores more than the mode of input.

Figure 2 compares the Visual Input scores (V-O & V-W) on the VADS

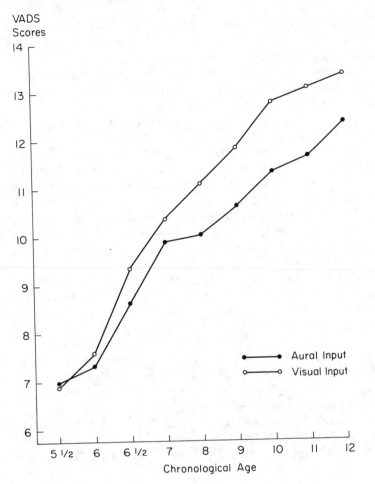

Figure 2. Comparison of aural and visual input scores.

Test with the Aural Input scores (A-O & A-W). It is shown that the discrepancy between the Aural and Visual Input scores increases as children get older, at least up to age 11. These results are consistent with the findings of other investigators (Carterette and Jones, 1967; Murray and Roberts, 1968; Senf, 1969). The consistently higher Visual Input scores do not necessarily reflect better visual perception or visual memory on the part of the youngsters. The difference between the Visual and Aural Input scores on the VADS seems to result from the fact that most school-age children verbalize the digits, either vocally or subvocally, when they read them. Thus, they use both visual and auditory cues when recalling visually presented digits. The visual presentation of digits also lends itself better to rehearsal than the auditory presentation of the digits (Corballis and Loveless, 1967).

The recall of aurally presented digits depends almost entirely on oral recall. It is rare for children to visualize digits as they hear them. As mentioned earlier, one occasionally finds youngsters who will write digits with their fingers on the table or in the air while listening to them; these children use their kinesthetic sense to help them in the recall of aurally presented digit sequences.

Based on the findings on Table 7 and Figure 2, one can expect elementary school pupils to have somewhat higher Visual Input scores than Aural Input scores. If the Aural Input and Visual Input scores are the same, one might suspect that the youngster is either still immature or that he has some difficulty with visual processing or recall strategies. When a child's Visual Input score is actually lower than the Aural Input score, then the pupil is most likely extremely immature or has serious problems in visual processing and visual memory. Just how significant a problem a child has in either Aural or Visual Input can only be determined by comparing his VADS Test scores with the mean and standard deviation scores on Table 7 or the percentile score on Table 8 (Appendix A) for his age level.

The fact that pupils process and recall visually presented symbols better than auditorily presented symbols has also practical implications for the instruction of first- to sixth-graders. It seems highly desirable that teachers use a multisensory approach, using both visual and auditory materials when introducing new lessons, especially if the pupils are expected to recall and to reproduce the material at a later date. Lectures without visual illustrations are apt to be less well remembered than illustrated lectures.

A meaningful assessment of a VADS Test score must always take the child's age into consideration. If an 8-year-old pupil obtains a Total VADS Test score of 21, then his VADS Test performance is average for his age group; but if the child were only 6 years old, rather than 8 years old, then his score of 21 would be outstanding; on the other hand if the youngster was 12 years old then a Total VADS Test score of 21 would be extremely poor. A given VADS Test score by itself has little meaning unless it is used with the normative tables.

PERCENTILE SCORES BY AGE LEVELS

Table 8 (Appendix A) shows the VADS Test percentile scores for children age 5½ to 12. This table was designed for the practicing clinician or diagnostician who wants more detailed information about a youngster's relative standing on the VADS Test than can be provided by the mean scores and standard deviations.

Plus/minus one standard deviation encompasses 68% of a given sample and extends from the 16th to the 84th percentile. A score of more than one S.D. from the mean can be regarded as very good, a score of less than one S.D. as very poor. Table 8 (Appendix A) gives the values for the 10th percentile, the 25th percentile, the 50th percentile or median, the 75th percentile, and the 90th percentile of the 11 VADS Test measures for each age level. Children whose VADS Test scores fall at or above the 90th percentile are considered outstanding on that particular task; those with scores at the 75th percentile are high average on the VADS Test; those with scores at the 50th percentile or Median are average; scores at the 25th percentile can be regarded as low average; whereas scores at or below the 10th percentile are thought to be very low or defective.

The VADS Test Combination scores (A I, V I, O E, W E, Intra, Inter) and the Total VADS score differentiate well between outstanding, high average, average, low average, and very low performances of children age 5½ to 10; thereafter the VADS Test scores can no longer discriminate between high average and exceptionally good performances because the ceiling of the VADS Test is relatively low. Since the required task is comparatively easy, one fourth of the 11- and 12-year-old youngsters of the normative sample had perfect or near perfect scores on the VADS Test. However, the VADS Test scores can differentiate effectively between average and below average test performances not only of younger children but also of fifth- and sixth-graders.

For example, if an 11-year-old pupil has a Visual Input score (V I) of 14, one can only say with certainty that his score is at least average; one cannot state whether his performance is average, high average, or outstanding. On the other hand, if an 11-year-old has a Visual Input score of 11, then it is safe to assume that his visual processing and his recall of visually presented symbols is extremely poor since the score of 11 falls below the 10th percentile for 11-year-old pupils.

The situation is somewhat different for the four VADS Subtests (A-O, V-O, A-W, V-W) since their range of scores is so limited. It can be seen on Table 8 that a given score may frequently be either very low (10th percentile) or low average (25th percentile), or a score may be average (50th percentile) as well as high average (75th percentile), and so on. For instance, an Aural-Oral score of 3 would be considered low (10th percentile) for 5½- and 6-year-old children, but a Visual-Oral score of 3 would not necessarily be a very poor score for kindergarten pupils since this test score could be either very low (10th percentile) or low average (25th percentile). Only a Visual-Oral score of 2 can be thought of as defective for 5½- and 6-year-olds.

Table 8 shows that for 7-year-old children, Aural-Written scores of 4, 5, and 6 are all within the average range, from the 25th to the 75th percentile, but a score of 4 is also very poor (10th percentile) and a score of 6 is also very good (90th percentile). In this case only a score of less than 4 can be thought of as defective and only a score of 7 can be regarded as truly outstanding.

TOTAL VADS SCORES AND AGE EQUIVALENTS

When assessing a Total VADS Test score of a very immature or educationally handicapped child, it is not only helpful to compare his Total VADS Test score with the Total VADS Test scores of other children of his age level but also to know what actual age level his VADS Test performance is on. If, for instance, a 10-year-old pupil obtains a Total VADS Test score of 20, one can say that his VADS Test performance is at the 10th percentile for 10-year-old children (Table 8), and that it resembles the performance of 7½-year-old youngsters. Table 9 (Appendix B) shows the Total VADS Test scores and their age equivalents.

MEANS AND STANDARD DEVIATIONS BY GRADE LEVEL

The VADS Test has particular value as a screening test for school beginners and as a diagnostic test for children with learning difficulties. For this reason, it is important to provide grade level norms for the VADS Test in addition to age level normative data. Table 10 gives the VADS Test means and standard deviations for each grade level from the end of kindergarten through the sixth grade. The data were derived from the VADS Test records of 656 public school pupils who were part of the normative sample. These youngsters represented a socioeconomic and ethnic cross section.

The grade level mean scores are, of course, similar to the VADS Test scores for the different age levels, shown on Table 7. There was a steady improvement on the VADS Test scores from one grade level to the next, but the greatest improvements were revealed between the end- of-kindergarten and the first-grade scores, and between the first- and second-grade scores. As previously mentioned, both maturation in perceptual-motor integration and the learning of recall strategies and writing skills contribute to the marked gain in VADS Test scores between the ages of 5½ and 7. Thereafter the change in VADS Test scores is much more gradual. It is not certain if the VADS Test scores of seventh-graders are better than the VADS Test scores of sixth-graders. This study only included pupils up to the sixth grade. However, for slowly maturing, vulnerable youngsters with learning difficulties the VADS Test scores continue to improve up to age 14 and possibly longer (see Chapter 9).

Table 10 shows that the Visual Input (V-O & V-W) scores for the various grade levels, starting with the first grade, were markedly higher than the Aural Input (A-O & A-W) scores. The Visual and Aural Input scores differed only slightly for the end-of-kindergarten pupils. There were no consistent differences on Table 10 between the scores for Oral and Written Expression or between the scores for Intrasensory and Intersensory Integration.

A number of other investigators administered the VADS Test to groups of first-, second-, third-, fourth-, and fifth-graders. Table 11 compares the VADS Test mean scores they obtained with the normative data. Also shown on this table are the mean scores from an earlier study (Koppitz, 1970) with well-functioning, middle-class pupils, and the VADS Test means of entire public school classes, from lower- and lower-middle-income backgrounds, that I tested while collecting normative data.

As would be expected, Table 11 reveals some variations between the VADS Test means scores of different socioeconomic groups. For this reason, I would suggest that school psychologists establish their own VADS Test norms for the youngsters in their school district, so that they can compare a given pupil's performance to that of other children of his grade level. This is

Table 10.

VADS Test Mean Scores and Standard Deviations for Grades K to 6

VADS	Kindergarten (N 160)			1st Grade (N 94)			2nd Grade (N 121)			3rd Grade (N 85)		
	Mean	S.D.	±1 S.D.	Mean	S.D.	±1 S.D.	Mean	S.D.	±1 S.D.	Mean	S.D.	±1 S.D.
A-O	4.1	.83	3.3–4.9	4.7	.88	3.8–5.6	5.2	.88	4.3–6.1	5.4	.90	4.5–6.3
V-O	4.0	1.19	2.8–5.2	5.0	.87	4.1–5.9	5.5	1.02	4.5–6.5	5.8	1.00	4.8–6.8
A-W	3.0	1.10	1.9–4.1	4.4	.92	3.5–5.3	4.8	.90	3.9–5.7	5.0	.92	4.1–5.9
V-W	3.4	1.29	3.1–4.7	4.7	.89	3.8–5.6	5.4	.96	4.4–6.4	5.8	1.05	4.8–6.9
A I	7.2	1.70	5.5–8.9	9.1	1.53	7.6–10.6	10.0	1.53	8.5–11.5	10.4	1.59	9.0–12.0
V I	7.4	2.29	5.1–9.7	9.8	1.50	8.3–11.3	10.9	1.79	9.1–12.7	11.6	1.81	9.8–13.4
O E	8.1	1.77	6.3–9.9	9.8	1.50	8.3–11.3	10.6	1.53	9.1–12.1	11.2	1.52	9.7–12.7
W E	6.4	2.26	4.1–8.7	9.1	1.56	7.5–10.7	10.3	1.53	8.8–11.8	10.9	1.64	9.3–12.5
Intra	7.5	2.21	5.3–9.7	9.5	1.47	8.0–11.0	10.6	1.46	9.1–12.1	11.2	1.60	9.6–12.8
Inter	7.0	2.12	4.9–9.1	9.4	1.49	7.9–10.9	10.3	1.59	8.7–11.9	10.8	1.56	9.2–12.4
Total	14.5	3.77	10.8–18.3	18.9	2.70	16.2–21.6	20.9	2.80	18.1–23.7	22.0	2.88	19.1–24.9

VADS	4th Grade (N 69)			5th Grade (N 88)			6th Grade (N 48)		
	Mean	S.D.	±1 S.D.	Mean	S.D.	±1 S.D.	Mean	S.D.	±1 S.D.
A-O	5.7	.92	4.8–6.6	5.9	.94	5.0–6.8	6.1	.90	5.2–7.0
V-O	6.4	.86	5.5–7.3	6.5	.73	5.8–7.2	6.7	.57	6.1–7.3
A-W	5.5	.99	4.5–6.5	5.5	1.08	4.4–6.6	6.1	.98	5.1–7.1
V-W	6.3	.94	5.4–7.2	6.6	.64	6.0–7.2	6.8	.64	6.2–7.4
A I	11.2	1.73	9.5–12.9	11.4	1.78	9.6–13.2	12.2	1.62	10.6–13.8
V I	12.6	1.51	10.1–14.1	13.0	1.13	11.9–14.1	13.5	1.11	12.4–14.6
O E	12.0	1.48	10.5–13.5	12.3	1.39	10.9–13.7	12.8	1.32	11.5–14.1
W E	11.8	1.55	10.3–13.4	12.1	1.54	10.6–13.6	12.8	1.42	11.4–14.2
Intra	12.0	1.53	10.5–13.5	12.4	1.33	11.1–13.7	12.8	1.34	11.5–14.1
Inter	11.8	1.57	10.2–13.4	11.9	1.56	10.3–13.5	12.8	1.34	11.5–14.1
Total	23.8	2.80	21.0–26.6	24.4	2.65	21.8–27.1	25.6	2.50	23.1–28.1

Table 11.

VADS Test Scores by Grade Level

Examiner	Grade	N	Socioeconomic	VADS Test Mean Scores				
				A–O	V–O	A–W	V–W	Total
Normative	K	160	cross section	4.11	3.99	3.04	3.36	14.50
Koppitz	K	24	middle class	4.3	4.3	3.4	3.4	15.4
Normative	1st	94	cross section	4.73	5.03	4.39	4.65	18.87
Koppitz	1st	20	middle class, high achiever	5.00	5.45	5.00	5.15	20.60
Hurd	1st	12	middle class	5.08	5.33	4.42	4.92	19.75
Koppitz	1st	24	lower class	4.33	4.75	3.83	4.12	17.04
Normative	2nd	112	cross section	5.09	5.47	4.85	5.42	20.82
Hurd	2nd	40	middle class, high IQ	5.17	5.90	5.00	5.85	21.93
Hurd	2nd	12	middle class	5.25	5.75	4.92	5.92	21.84
Koppitz	2nd	20	middle class, high achiever	4.90	5.95	4.85	5.80	21.50
Rubin	2nd	32	upper middle class	5.44	5.31	4.84	5.00	20.59
Koppitz	2nd	24	lower middle class	5.08	5.13	4.75	5.33	20.29
Baldwin	2nd	20	upper middle class	4.80	6.05	4.50	5.05	19.90
Rubin	2nd	30	lower class	5.03	4.77	4.90	4.67	19.37
Rubin	2nd	31	lower middle class	5.32	4.65	4.61	4.42	19.00
Witkin	2nd	272	lower to middle	4.77	4.97	4.41	4.70	18.85
Rubin	2nd	39	middle class	4.97	4.67	4.38	4.41	18.43
Normative	3rd	85	cross section	5.39	5.78	5.04	5.81	22.01
Morea	3rd	43	upper middle class	5.40	5.98	5.47	6.23	23.08
Koppitz	3rd	20	middle class, high achiever	5.14	5.75	5.10	6.00	22.00
Koppitz	3rd	25	low to middle class	5.28	5.92	4.84	5.80	21.84
Hurd	3rd	12	middle class	5.33	5.83	4.83	5.83	21.82
Normative	4th	69	cross section	5.69	6.35	5.48	6.28	23.78
Carr	4th	26	middle class	5.9	6.7	6.0	6.6	25.3
Koppitz	4th	20	middle class, high achiever	6.00	6.45	6.10	6.50	25.05
Hurd	4th	12	middle class	5.50	6.42	5.25	6.17	23.34
Normative	5th	88	cross section	5.89	6.45	5.49	6.59	24.40
Koppitz	5th	20	middle class, high achiever	6.15	6.65	6.10	6.75	25.65
Koppitz	5th	27	lower-middle class	6.04	6.37	5.52	6.59	24.52
Hurd	5th	12	middle class	5.92	6.92	5.58	6.42	24.50
Normative	6th	48	cross section	6.08	6.73	6.06	6.75	25.62

especially important when the VADS Test, or any other test, is used for screening purposes.

PERCENTILE SCORES BY GRADE LEVEL

Table 12 (Appendix C) shows the percentile scores for grades 1 to 6 and for end-of-kindergarten pupils. The 10th, 25th, 50th, 75th, and 90th percentiles scores are given for each of the grade levels. The interpretation of the percentile scores is the same as for the percentile scores for different age levels (Table 8) as previously discussed. The data on Table 12 are especially useful when trying to establish a given child's functioning level on the VADS Test in relation to other youngsters of the same grade level.

The VADS Test Combination scores (A I, V I, O E, W E, Intra, and Inter) discriminate well between very low, low average, average, high average, and outstanding test performances of kindergarten to fourth-grade pupils. For fifth- and sixth-graders, the VADS Test Combination scores can assess very low to high average performance, but they are not able to differentiate between high average and outstanding pupils. Children who obtain a perfect score of 14, as many of the better fifth- and sixth-graders are apt to do, can no longer improve their test scores.

The Total VADS Test scores discriminate best, of all the VADS Test measures, between the various functioning levels for all grades, from kindergarten to the sixth grade. As was pointed out previously, the four VADS Subtests (A-O, V-O, A-W, V-W) have a very limited score range and are, therefore, usually only able to differentiate between high, low, and average test performances of elementary school children. Because of this, it is recommended that the VADS Test Combination scores and the Total VADS Test score be primarily considered when using Table 12 to assess a given youngster's VADS Test performance.

NORMATIVE DATA: SUMMARY

The normative data for the VADS Test were derived from 810 public school pupils who represented a socioeconomic cross section. No significant differences were found between the VADS Test scores of boys and girls. VADS Test norms were provided for children age 5½ to 12, and for pupils from kindergarten through the sixth grade. In addition, age equivalents were given for Total VADS Test scores.

Chapter 8

VADS Test and School Achievement

The VADS Test was designed as a diagnostic test for children with learning difficulties. The question that presents itself is, therefore: How close is the relationship between VADS Test scores and school achievement? This chapter explores three different aspects of the relationship between the achievement of public school pupils and their performance on VADS Tests. First we consider the effectiveness of the VADS Test as a long-term predictor of school achievement; then the correlation between VADS Test scores and achievement scores, obtained at the same time, is determined; finally a comparison is made between the VADS Test performance of average public school pupils and of youngsters with learning problems.

PREDICTING SCHOOL ACHIEVEMENT

In the process of collecting normative data for the VADS Test, I tested 100 kindergarten pupils during the last month of the school year. Three years later I was able to locate the school records of 46 of these youngsters shortly after they had been given the Comprehensive Test of Basic Skills or CTBS (1973). With a few exceptions all of the 46 children were white, middle-class, and of at least average mental ability. The mean CTBS IQ score for the group was 111.5 with an IQ range from 82 to 144. Only three of the youngsters had IQ scores of less than 90. However, it must be recognized that the CTBS tends to score relatively high at the third-grade level and that the test scores should be regarded with caution. The 46 children in this study obtained, at the end of third grade, the following mean grade level scores on the CTBS: Total Reading 5.44, Total Language 6.09, Total Arithmetic 5.03, and Total Battery 5.45.

When I administered the VADS Test to the 100 youngsters in kindergarten, three of them were unable to read and write any digits. One of these three children was transferred two years later to a special class for children with learning disabilities; the other two were among the third-grade pupils here under discussion. These two children were both functioning at the end-of-first to beginning second-grade level on the CTBS, that is, they tested about four grade levels below the average of the group as a whole.

Chi-squares were computed comparing the youngsters with CTBS Total Reading and Total Battery scores of 4.6 or above, and those with scores of 4.5 or less; and those with Total Language and Total Arithmetic scores of 5.0 and higher with those who scored 4.9 or less. The youngsters were also divided according to whether they scored on the 11 VADS Test measures above the 25th percentile or at or below the 25th percentile. The percentile scores were derived from Table 8. Table 13 shows the Chi-square values and the level of significance when comparing the 11 VADS Test scores, obtained at the end of kindergarten, with third-grade achievement on the CTBS for the 46 youngsters.

The results on Table 13 indicate that the VADS Test, administered at the end of kindergarten, is an effective predictor of third-grade achievement, as measured on the CTBS. Although all four CTBS measures investigated were found to be closely related to the VADS Test scores of school beginners, the VADS Test seems to be most closely related to Language skills, including language mechanics, expression, and spelling.

Among the various VADS Test scores that were obtained in kindergarten, the ones most closely associated with third-grade achievement on the CTBS were the Aural Input, Intrasensory Integration, and Intersensory Integration scores. It was particularly noteworthy that the Aural-Oral and Visual-Written Subtests, and the Aural Input and Intersensory Integration scores, all showed a high correlation with third-grade reading. As shown in the following, these particular VADS Test measures were not related to reading when the VADS Test scores and the CTBS Scores were both obtained at the fifth-grade level. It is important, therefore, to take children's ages into consideration when using the VADS Test as a predictive or diagnostic instrument.

Since many kindergarten pupils are still unsure about reading and writing digits, it was not surprising that the Visual Input and Written Expression scores of kindergarten pupils were relatively less able to predict third grade achievement than the Aural Input and Oral Expression scores.

The findings of this study and my experience with school beginners have convinced me that the VADS Test is a valuable addition to a screening battery for end-of-kindergarten or beginning first-grade pupils. An analysis of the Total VADS Test scores revealed that, with a few exceptions, kindergarten youngsters who scored above the 25th percentile had at least average or better CTBS scores in the third grade; whereas, the majority, but not all, of the children who scored at or below the 25th percentile, at the end of kindergarten, had below average third-grade achievement on the CTBS. Children who were unable to complete the VADS Test at the end of kindergarten were also poor students 3 years later.

Even though the VADS Test appears to be able to predict achievement in the third grade, it should not be used by itself as a screening instrument; nor should any other brief test or measure, for that matter. The achievement of any given pupil depends on a combination and interaction of various mental, social, emotional, and physical factors. A meaningful screening battery has to take as many of these factors as possible into consideration. The VADS Test taps only a limited number of them. Chapter 15 describes a brief screening battery for end-of-kindergarten or beginning first-grade pupils that I have found useful (Koppitz, 1975a, p. 99).

Table 13.

Kindergarten VADS and Third-Grade Achievement on the CTBS

VADS	Total Reading		Total Language		Total Arithmetic		Total Battery	
	χ^2	p	χ^2	p	χ^2	p	χ^2	p
A–O	8.15	.01	4.14	.05	6.93	.01	10.33	.01
V–O	4.41	.05	10.45	.01	3.55	.05	5.92	.05
A–W	4.73	.05	15.96	.001	not significant		8.15	.01
V–W	8.98	.01	12.00	.001	5.99	.05	10.43	.01
A I	11.64	.001	8.86	.01	9.82	.01	14.93	.001
V I	4.41	.05	7.99	.01	3.55	.05	5.92	.05
O E	7.55	.01	8.86	.01	6.11	.05	10.15	.01
W E	not significant		5.64	.05	not significant		4.29	.05
Intra	10.06	.01	10.45	.01	8.61	.01	12.66	.001
Inter	8.15	.01	13.10	.001	6.93	.01	10.33	.01
Total	5.49	.05	10.96	.001	6.30	.01	8.86	.01

VADS TEST AND ACHIEVEMENT SCORES

The preceding section discussed the ability of the VADS Test, administered at the end of kindergarten, to predict achievement three years in the future. This section explores the correlation between VADS Test performance and school achievement when both measures are obtained at the same time. Information about this relationship was derived from six different studies.

The first of these was part of a major project on "Reading Improvement through Auditory Perceptual Training." This investigation, as reported by Witkin (1971), used 272 second-grade pupils as subjects. The youngsters were given a comprehensive battery of tests; later all of the tests were correlated with each other. Among the tests that were administered were the four VADS Subtests and the Comprehension section of the Gilmore Oral Reading Test (1968).

There is little reason to expect a reading comprehension test to correlate with a test of perceptual-motor processing, sequencing, and recall, yet Witkin found a statistically significant ($p < .01$) relationship between the Visual-Oral and Visual-Written Subtests and reading comprehension. The correlations for all four Subtests were: Aural-Oral: $r = .18$, Visual-Oral: $r = .35$, Aural-Written: $r = .14$, and Visual-Written: $r = .25$. Of the four Subtests, the Visual-Oral Subtest was most closely related to reading. This is consistent with the results of a recent study (Koppitz, 1975b) in which the Visual-Oral Subtest differentiated best between 8- and 9-year-old readers and nonreaders.

Shumar (1976) and Thompson (1976) correlated the four VADS Subtest scores and the Total VADS Test scores with the reading scores of the Peabody Individual Achievement Test (PIAT) (Dunn and Markwardt, 1970) and the California Achievement Test (CAT) (Tiegs and Clark, 1970) of second-, third-, fourth-, and fifth-graders. All the children were of average mental ability and came from a low socioeconomic, rural background. The four groups included from 18 to 29 pupils each.

The results of the two studies showed that Reading Recognition on the PIAT was related to the VADS Test performance of the second-, third- and fourth-graders, but not to that of the fifth-graders. PIAT Reading Comprehension was only related to the Aural-Written and Visual-Written scores of the second-graders. On the CAT the Reading Vocabulary scores correlated significantly with some of the VADS Test scores at all four grade levels tested. The CAT Reading Comprehension and Total Reading scores were significantly associated with some of the VADS Test scores of the second-, fourth- and fifth-graders, but not with the VADS Test scores of the third-graders.

For the second-graders the Aural-Written, Visual-Written, and Total VADS Test scores were most closely related to the PIAT and CAT reading scores; for the third-graders the Aural-Oral, Visual-Oral, and Total VADS Test scores correlated best with the reading scores. At the fourth-grade level the Visual-Oral and Visual-Written Subtest scores were most closely associated with the reading measures, whereas fifth-grade Aural-Oral, Visual-Oral, Visual-Written, and Total VADS Test scores correlated significantly with the CAT reading scores but not with the PIAT reading scores. It thus appears that the Visual-Oral and Visual-Written Subtests and the Total VADS Test scores were most closely related to reading achievement on the PIAT and CAT.

Hurd (1971) examined the ability of the VADS Test to distinguish between high achieving and low achieving middle-class pupils. Her subjects were divided into two groups. Group A included 12 first-graders, 12 second-graders, and 12 third-graders. Of these, 18 children were functioning at the top fourth of their classes and the other 18 youngsters were at the bottom of their respective classes according to teacher ratings. Group B included 12 good- and 12 low-functioning fourth- and fifth-grade pupils. Using Fisher's t statistic, Hurd found significant differences ($p < .05$) between the high and low achievers in Group A on the Aural-Oral, Aural-Written, and Visual-Written Subtests, and on the Aural Input, Visual Input, Oral Expression, Written Expression and Intersensory Integration scores. Hurd did not use the Intrasensory Integration or the Total VADS Test scores. With Group B, only the Visual-Oral Subtest and the Intersensory Integration scores were able to distinguish between the good and poor students.

Hurd's study offers strong support for the hypothesis that most of the VADS Test measures are related to school achievement in the primary grades. For middle-class fourth- and fifth-graders this relationship was limited to the Visual-Oral Subtest and to Intersensory Integration only. However, my own study with an entire class of fifth-graders showed very different results.

In the course of administering the VADS Test to the normative sample I tested an entire fifth grade in a school located in a lower- to lower-middle class neighborhood. The youngsters had been given the Comprehensive Test of Basic Skills (CTBS) (1973) just a few days earlier. The 26 children had an age mean of 11–0 years and ranged in mental ability from superior to borderline. Using the Chi-square statistic I compared the 11 VADS Test measures with the following CTBS scores: Total Reading, Total Language, Spelling, Total Arithmetic, Total Battery, Total IQ score. Table 14 reveals how the VADS Test scores and the CTBS scores were dichotomized, and the resulting Chi-square and p values.

According to Table 14 there was a significant relationship among 9 of the 11 VADS Test measures and the Spelling and Total Language scores of the CTBS. The Total Arithmetic and Total Battery scores of the CTBS were closely related to 8 of the VADS Test measures. The CTBS Total Reading score measures mainly reading comprehension and vocabulary, these functions are not measured by the VADS Test. It is therefore not surprising that the CTBS Total Reading score correlated significantly with only four of the VADS Test measures (V-O, O E, Intra, Total VADS). The CTBS Total IQ score was found to correlate significantly with the Visual-Written. Visual Input, Oral Expression, Intrasensory Integration and the Total VADS Test scores.

Table 14.
Fifth-Grade VADS Test and CTBS Achievement Scores

VADS (Hi/Lo)	Total Readings (5.5-/5.4-)		Total Language (6.0-/5.9-)		Spelling (5.5-/5.4-)		Total Arithmetic (5.6-/5.5-)		Total Battery (6.0-/5.9-)		Total IQ (95-/94-)	
	χ^2	p	χ^2	p	χ^2	p	χ^2	p	χ^2	p	χ^2	p
A–O (7/6)	not significant		not significant		not significant		not significant		not significant		not significant	
V–O (7/6)	3.87	.05	5.67	.05	10.08	.01	5.67	.05	5.67	.05	not significant	
A–W (6/5)	not significant		not significant		5.67	.05	not significant		not significant		not significant	
V–W (7/6)	not significant		7.62	.01	7.62	.01	not significant		3.71	.05	3.76	.05
A I (12/11)	not significant		5.67	.05	not significant		5.67	.05	5.67	.05	not significant	
V I (14/13)	not significant		7.39	.01	12.40	.001	4.21	.05	3.72	.05	3.87	.05
O E (14/13)	7.05	.01	10.08	.01	10.08	.01	10.08	.01	10.08	.08	3.87	.05
W E (13/12)	not significant		3.72	.05	7.43	.01	not significant		not significant		not significant	
Intra (14/13)	4.06	.05	9.27	.01	4.96	.05	3.43	.05	4.96	.05	5.44	.05
Inter (13/12)	not significant		3.72	.05	7.43	.01	4.21	.05	3.72	.05	not significant	
Total (24/23)	6.12	.05	3.27	.05	7.62	.01	5.05	.05	7.62	.01	3.76	.05

A further analysis of the findings on Table 14 shows that the Visual-Oral and Visual-Written Subtests are more closely associated with fifth-grade achievement than are the Aural-Oral and Aural-Written Subtests. Particularly interesting is the fact that Aural-Oral Subtest scores that had high predictive value at the kindergarten level showed no statistically significant relationship to any of the six CTBS measures at the fifth-grade level. The highest correlations between the VADS Test performance and achievement of the fifth-graders occurred with the Visual-Oral Subtest and with the Visual Input, Oral Expression, Intrasensory and Intersensory Integration, and Total VADS Test scores. The Written Expression score was mainly related to spelling.

The Visual-Written Subtest and the Visual Input, Oral Expression, Intrasensory Integration, and Total VADS Test scores were also significantly related to the CTBS IQ scores. A child's mental ability obviously affects his performance on the VADS Test to a certain extent. As was mentioned previously, brighter children tend to use more effective strategies for the processing and recall of digit sequences. Yet Table 14 clearly shows that the VADS Test scores of fifth-graders were more closely related to their achievement than to their IQ scores.

The VADS Test measures the mechanics of learning, such as perceptual-motor integration, sequencing, and recall; these mechanics are essential for school achievement. Most youngsters of average mental ability can master them without effort, but children with learning disabilities often have problems in the area of perceptual-motor integration and recall, even when their abstract reasoning ability is within the average range. On the other hand, some rather dull children, with poor reasoning ability, may have good memory for symbol sequences and facts (Koppitz, 1971, p. 110; Spitz and Lafontaine, 1973). The relationship between the VADS Test and IQ scores is discussed more fully in Chapter 12.

VADS TEST OF CHILDREN WITH AND WITHOUT LEARNING DISABILITIES

The preceding sections demonstrated that the VADS Test is related to the achievement of normal public school pupils. At this time we compare the VADS Test scores of average schoolchildren with the VADS Test scores of youngsters with serious learning difficulties.

Baldwin (1976) examined the Total VADS Test score and the Reading and Spelling scores on the Wide Range Achievement Test (Jastack et al., 1965) of two groups of upper middle-class second-grade pupils. Group I consisted of 20 students who were rated "average" by their teachers, whereas Group II was made up of 20 pupils who were referred to Resource Rooms because of learning disabilities. The test score means for the two groups were as follows:

Mean Scores	Group I	Group II
Slosson IQ	115	108
Total VADS Test	19.9	17.9
Reading Recognition	4.0	2.3
Spelling	3.5	2.3

Spearman Rankorder correlations between the WRAT Reading and Spelling scores and the Total VADS Test scores were not statistically significant for the average pupils in Group I. The learning-disabled youngsters in Group II showed a highly significant relationship between the Total VADS Test and the Reading scores ($r = .62$, $p < .01$). The correlation between the Spelling scores and the Total VADS Test scores was positive but not statistically significant ($r = .36$, $p. < .10$).

In an earlier study (Koppitz, 1973) I compared, by means of Chi-squares, the VADS Subtest scores of 32 boys with emotional and learning problems with the VADS Subtest scores of 20 average public school pupils. The two groups of youngsters were matched for sex and age (C.A. 9–0 to 10–11). All of the children were of at least average mental ability. The control group was found to have significantly higher VADS Test scores than the learning-disabled youngsters on three of the Subtests: Visual-Oral $\chi^2 = 7.1$, $p < .01$; Aural-Written $\chi^2 = 3.5$, $p < .05$; Visual-Written $\chi^2 = 11.7$, $p < .001$. Only the Aural-Oral Subtest failed to differentiate between the two groups of children.

In another study (Koppitz, 1975b), it was shown that the VADS Test could differentiate between a group of 23 children with serious learning problems and a control group of 30 average pupils. The youngsters were matched for sex, age (C.A. 8–1 to 9–11), and WISC IQ scores (IQ range 91 to 118). In this investigation, the Chi-square values for all four VADS Subtests were highly significant; Aural-Oral $\chi^2 = 14.2$, $p < .001$; Visual-Oral $\chi^2 = 20.5$, $p < .001$; Aural-Written $\chi^2 = 8.9$, $p < .01$; Visual-Written $\chi^2 = 15.8$, $p < .001$; Total VADS Test $\chi^2 = 22.7$, $p < .001$.

During the process of collecting normative data for the VADS Test, I administered the test to an entire second grade, third grade, and fifth grade in a school located in a lower- to lower-middle-class neighborhood. Later I was able to match the 22 second-graders, the 24 third-graders, and the 27 fifth-graders with special class pupils with learning disabilities to whom I had also administered the VADS Test. The two groups of youngsters were paired and matched for exact age, sex, socio-ethnic background, and mental ability. No retarded, severely disturbed, or physically handicapped children were included in the study.

Chi-squares were computed comparing the average pupils and the learning-disabled children whose VADS Test scores were above the 25th percentile with those whose VADS Test scores were at or below the 25th percentile. The percentile scores were derived from Table 8 (Appendix A). Table 15 shows the Chi-square values obtained and their level of significance.

The results of all three grade levels and for all 11 VADS Test scores were statistically significant. The children with learning disabilities scored

Table 15.
Comparison of VADS Test Scores of Normal and LD Pupils

VADS	Second-Graders		Third-Graders		Fifth-Graders	
	χ^2	p	χ^2	p	χ^2	p
A–O	20.62	.001	15.19	.001	16.88	.001
V–O	7.49	.01	10.15	.01	6.75	.01
A–W	10.11	.01	4.20	.05	5.20	.05
V–W	20.45	.001	5.58	.05	12.96	.001
A I	23.32	.001	5.83	.05	8.98	.01
V I	21.15	.001	8.35	.01	9.08	.01
O E	18.79	.001	18.88	.001	16.88	.001
W E	14.57	.001	8.35	.01	9.28	.01
Intra	23.71	.001	12.54	.001	14.60	.001
Inter	10.92	.001	10.15	.01	4.99	.05
Total	18.79	.001	10.76	.001	12.53	.001

markedly lower on the VADS Test than the average pupils in the second, third, and fourth grades.

Obviously, not every child with learning disabilities will have difficulties with each of the 11 VADS Test measures, nor is perceptual-motor integration, sequencing, and recall, as measured on the VADS Test, necessarily the main cause of learning problems in children. But the results of the four studies discussed above show that the VADS Test is a useful diagnostic instrument for learning problems in elementary school pupils.

VADS TEST AND SCHOOL ACHIEVEMENT: SUMMARY

The VADS Test, administered to pupils at the end of kindergarten, was able to predict third-grade achievement on the CTBS. It appears that for young children the Aural-Oral, Aural-Written, and Aural Input scores have particular diagnostic significance, whereas for second- to fifth-grade pupils the Visual-Oral, Visual-Written, and Visual Input scores are more closely related to achievement, especially to reading achievement. All VADS Test scores were able to differentiate between high- and low-achieving elementary school children, and they could discriminate significantly between normal public school pupils and youngsters with serious learning disabilities.

Chapter 9

The VADS Test and Learning Difficulties

The preceding chapters discussed the VADS Test performance of groups of normal public school children and its relationship to achievement. It was also shown that the VADS Test scores of groups of average pupils differ significantly from those of children with learning disabilities. At this time we explore in depth the VADS Test performance of learning-disabled and retarded youngsters age 6 to 14. For, as has been emphasized repeatedly, the VADS Test was primarily designed as a diagnostic instrument to help analyze children's learning difficulties and to assist with the prescription of individualized programs to help correct or minimize such problems.

The following investigations are based on 873 VADS Test records obtained over a 6-year period from 443 different children with learning difficulties and from 102 moderately retarded youngsters. This means that some pupils contributed more than one VADS Test record to these studies, but none contributed more than one record at any one age level. For example, I administered the VADS Test to Mary, a student with serious learning disabilities, at age 8, 9½, 10, 11½, 12½, and 13½. Thus, Mary is represented in the VADS Test sample of LD pupils for age 8, 9, 10, 11, 12, and 13.

I gave the VADS Test to almost all the pupils I saw for psychological evaluation in the special classes for learning-disabled youngsters and in the Resource Rooms. The children in the Resource Rooms were enrolled in regular classes. They only came to the Resource Rooms for one or two periods each day for special help because they were unable to cope with a regular reading, math, or social studies class. All of these youngsters were of normal mental potential, but they were functioning on such a low level that they required an alternative program or supportive help in one or two key subjects.

The special class students usually suffered from a combination of serious learning, emotional, and behavior problems. They needed more than just 1 or 2 hours of special help per day. These children were in need of small, highly structured, and supportive classes and of individualized instructions in most of their academic subjects. The youngsters' mental ability ranged from the superior to the moderately retarded level. With a few exceptions, all the youngsters attended special classes that were located in regular school buildings and the children were integrated into regular gym, art, and music classes and into those academic classes with which they could cope. A small number of the special class pupils were so disturbed that they had to be placed into special classes at the regional center where their needs could be better met.

The learning-disabled children in these investigations were divided into three groups (A, B, C) on the basis of their mental ability as measured on the WISC or WISC-R. Table 16 shows the distribution of the youngsters by age, sex, and IQ scores. The 331 children in Group A represented LD pupils with average or above average mental ability (IQ 90 or above); Group B includes 441 dull normal to borderline (IQ 70 to 89) children, whereas the remaining 131 youngsters in Group C were moderately retarded (IQ 69 to 52).

The three groups differed significantly in their ratio of boys to girls. For Group A the ratio of boys to girls was 1:5; for Group B the ratio was 3:2; for Group C the ratio was almost 1:1 with a slightly larger number of girls than boys. I have found this pattern of sex distribution among special class pupils with serious learning problems to be quite typical; more boys than girls are referred for special educational services and they tend to be brighter and also tend to have more emotional and behavior problems; the girls who are referred to special classes are more often mentally limited. Yet, when the boys and girls in Groups A, B, and C were matched for exact age and IQ scores there was no significant difference between their VADS Test scores. The VADS Test scores were compared by means of the Wilcoxen matched pairs signed-ranks test (Siegel, 1956). In view of these findings the learning-disabled (LD) and mentally retarded (MR) boys and girls are not discussed separately, but are treated as single groups at each age level.

At each age level, from age 6½ to 13 and 14 years, the VADS Test scores of the LD and MR youngsters are compared with the normative data (Table 7) and with the Bender Gestalt Test and IQ scores; and finally VADS Test score patterns related to specific types of learning problems are explored.

Table 17 to Table 24 show the characteristics of the LD and MR pupils. The achievement test scores, reported on the tables, were obtained from the Wide Range Achievement Test (WRAT). The reading, spelling, and arithmetic mean scores are shown for each age level to give a detailed picture of the average functioning of the LD and MR pupils. It should also be noted that

Table 16.

Distribution of LD and MR Pupils by Age, Sex, and IQ Scores

Age	Group A (IQ 90 above)			Group B (IQ 70–89)			Group C (IQ 69 below)		
	Boys	Girls	Total	Boys	Girls	Total	Boys	Girls	Total
6–6/6–11	8	1	9	5	4	9	—	—	—
7–0/7–11	23	6	29	19	11	30	2	5	7
8–0/8–11	43	8	51	44	28	72	11	8	19
9–0/9–11	60	10	70	47	26	73	10	8	18
10–0/10–11	47	7	54	44	28	72	12	11	23
11–0/11–11	33	8	41	34	27	61	9	13	22
12–0/12–11	30	7	37	19	22	41	7	9	16
13–0/14–11	32	8	40	31	22	53	12	14	26
Total	276	55	331	243	168	411	63	63	131
	83%	17%	100%	59%	41%	100%	48%	52%	100%

Table 17.

Characteristics of LD Pupils Age 6–6 to 6–11

	Group A	Group B	
Age Mean	6–8	6–9	
Test	Mean (Range)	Mean (Range)	
WISC FS IQ	100.0 (90–127)	77.0 (70–89)	
Bender Test	9.6 (4–13)	12.4 (7–16)	
WRAT			
Reading Recognition	1.6 (1.2–2.3)	.6 (.0–1.3)	
Spelling	1.5 (.8–2.3)	.6 (.0–1.2)	
Arithmetic	1.5 (.5–2.4)	.6 (.0–1.2)	
VADS			VADS Norms
A–O	4.00	3.67	4.56
V–O	4.00	2.12	4.81
A–W	2.67	.78	4.09
V–W	2.78	1.11	4.53
A I	6.67	4.45	8.66
V I	6.78	3.23	9.35
O E	8.00	5.79	9.39
W E	5.45	1.89	8.63
Intra	6.78	4.78	9.11
Inter	6.67	2.90	8.91
Total	13.45	7.68	18.03

the WRAT scores tend to be rather high and that the reading scores measure only reading recognition, not reading comprehension. Thus, a youngster with a reading score of 3.2 on the WRAT cannot be expected to read a third-grade book with comprehension; his independent reading level is most likely at the middle second-grade level. A WRAT reading score of 3.2 does mean, however, that the child is able to recognize or to sound out, often slowly and laboriously, single words on the beginning third-grade level. It should also be pointed out that many LD children function very unevenly. Some of them function fairly well in arithmetic for instance, but not in reading and spelling, or they might be able to read but have difficulty with spelling and arithmetic, and so on.

CHARACTERISTICS OF LD AND MR PUPILS

Age 6½ to 7

Table 17 shows the characteristics of the 6½-year-old LD pupils in Group A and Group B only. The 6½-year-old moderately retarded youngsters in Group C were too immature to cope with any academic work or with the VADS Test. Even in Group A and Group B the children were still very immature in all areas. On the Bender Gestalt and Wide Range Achievement Test Group A functioned on the preprimer level, or like end-of-kindergarten pupils; Group B was on the prereadiness level and resembled beginning kindergarten children.

Table 18 exhibits the characteristics of the 7-year-old LD and MR pupils. Group A was functioning on the Bender and WRAT like beginning first-grade pupils; the youngsters in Group B were on the readiness level; and the children in Group C were on the level of beginning kindergarten pupils.

Most of the 7-year-old children in Group C, and many of the 6½ and 7 year olds in Group B had difficulty with the reading and writing of digits on the VADS Test. Even some of the youngsters in Group A were still uncertain about the writing of digits. The 6½- and 7- year-old LD children therefore did much better with the oral recall of digits on the VADS Test than with the written reproduction of the digit sequences. The VADS performance of young LD children is more determined by the mode of expression than by the mode of presenting the digit sequences.

As a group, the 6½- and 7-year-old pupils with learning difficulties showed a marked lag in their development of perceptual-motor integration, sequencing, and recall, as measured on the VADS Test. Figure 3 and Figure 4 give a graphic comparison of the VADS Test scores of Groups A, B, and C and the normative scores for 6½- and 7-year-old children. It is significant that the VADS Test scores of both the 6½- and 7-year-old pupils in Group A lack the characteristic distribution shown by average pupils; from age 6½ on, groups of normal youngsters tend to score higher on the two VADS Subtests with visual input (Visual-Oral and Visual-Written) than on the two VADS Subtests with aural presentation (Aural-Oral and Aural-Written). For average

Table 18.

Characteristics of LD and MR Pupils Age 7–0 to 7–11

	Group A	Group B	Group C	
Age Mean	7–6	7–6	7–10	
Test	Mean (Range)	Mean (Range)	Mean (Range)	
WISC FS IQ	102.2 (91–131)	79.1 (70–89)	63.7 (57–67)	
Bender Test	7.5 (1–14)	10.1 (1–15)	12.2 (6–18)	
WRAT				
Reading Recognition	1.7 (.2–3.9)	1.1 (.1–1.9)	.7 (.1–1.9)	
Spelling	1.5 (.8–2.6)	1.0 (.0–1.7)	.8 (.0–1.4)	
Arithmetic	1.9 (.3–3.0	1.1 (.1–1.8)	.3 (.1–.6)	
VADS				VADS Norms
A–O	4.12	4.13	3.26	5.12
V–O	4.28	3.50	2.00	5.31
A–W	3.69	2.77	1.57	4.79
V–W	3.38	2.43	1.14	5.10
A I	7.90	6.90	4.86	9.91
V I	7.66	5.93	3.14	10.42
O E	8.48	7.63	5.29	10.42
W E	7.06	5.20	2.71	9.90
Intra	7.59	6.57	4.43	10.24
Inter	7.97	6.27	3.57	10.09
Total	15.55	12.83	8.00	20.32

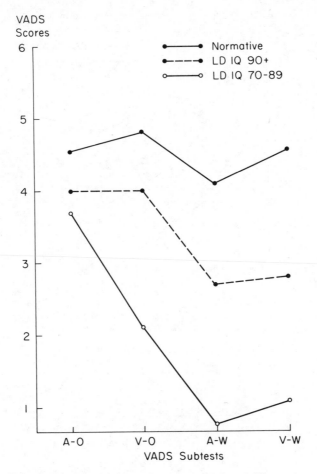

Figure 3. VADS Test mean scores—Age 6 1/2.

school-age children the mode of presenting the digits on the VADS Test is more important than the mode of expression.

The lower the mental ability of the children the more immature was their VADS Test performance. The 6½- and 7-year-old children in Group B performed less well on the VADS Test than the children in Group A and the VADS Test performance of the 7-year-old moderately retarded youngsters in Group C was markedly inferior to that of the 7-year-old pupils in Group B. For both Group B and Group C the Aural-Oral Subtest score was by far the highest because of the children's poor reading and writing ability.

This developmental lag usually has an organic basis and has to be taken into account when planning an educational program for young learning-disabled children. The causes for such a developmental lag may be manifold: Among the children in Groups A, B, and C were youngsters with medical histories of brain trauma and with diagnoses of brain lesions and neurological impairment; others were diagnosed as having "minimal brain dysfunction due to unknown causes"; others had histories of severe early deprivation and neglect; there were well-cared for, middle-class children

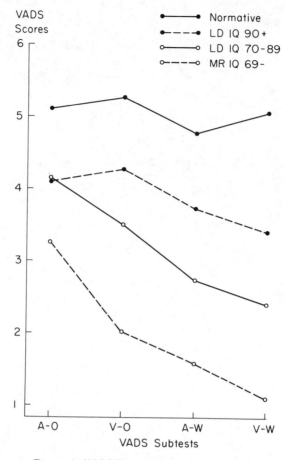

Figure 4. VADS Test mean scores—Age 7.

whose difficulties seemed to have a genetic basis and could be traced in familial patterns. Some youngsters had nothing "wrong" with them, they were merely slowly maturing children who were physically, mentally, emotionally, and socially immature for their age levels. A number of the LD and MR youngsters had suffered specific accidents or serious illnesses in early childhood. In this study the children were not grouped or analyzed on the basis of their diagnostic label but only according to their functioning level; a classroom teacher has to cope with youngsters' actual functioning and not with the diagnostic labels that have been given to the pupils. If a 7-year-old child has the maturation level of a kindergarten pupil, then he should be treated like a kindergarten child, regardless of what caused this immaturity.

Age 8 and 9

Table 19 and Table 20 show the characteristics of the LD and MR pupils ages 8 and 9. By age 8, the youngsters with normal mental ability in Group A were functioning on the end-of-first grade level; by age 9 they resembled

Table 19.
Characteristics of LD and MR Pupils Age 8–0 to 8–11

	Group A	Group B	Group C	
Age Mean	8–6	8–5	8–5	
Test	Mean (Range)	Mean (Range)	Mean (Range)	
WISC FS IQ	100.9 (90–137)	81.6 (72–89)	63.3 (54–68)	
Bender Test	5.5 (0–12)	9.1 (4–17)	11.7 (5–18)	
WRAT				
Reading Recognition	2.5 (1.1–7.0)	1.6 (.2–4.4)	1.2 (.6–1.4)	
Spelling	2.1 (.8–4.7)	1.5 (.1–3.0)	1.0 (.1–1.8)	
Arithmetic	2.0 (1.5–4.5)	1.8 (.3–3.0)	.9 (.2–1.8)	
VADS				VADS Norms
A–O	4.45	4.11	3.53	5.22
V–O	4.76	4.24	3.05	5.58
A–W	4.24	3.60	2.68	4.78
V–W	4.37	3.67	2.21	5.56
A I	8.75	7.68	6.21	10.00
V I	9.33	7.89	5.26	11.14
O E	9.25	8.36	6.58	10.80
W E	8.22	7.26	4.89	10.34
Intra	9.06	7.78	5.74	10.78
Inter	9.06	7.83	5.74	10.35
Total	18.12	15.61	11.47	21.14

Table 20.
Characteristics of LD and MR Pupils Age 9–0 to 9–11

	Group A	Group B	Group C	
Age Mean	9–6	9–5	9–5	
Test	Mean (Range)	Mean (Range)	Mean (Range)	
WISC FS IQ	99.5 (90–135)	80.9 (70–89)	63.1 (51–69)	
Bender Test	3.9 (0–12)	6.8 (1–14)	12.7 (5–18)	
WRAT				
Reading Recognition	2.7 (1.2–6.3)	2.0 (.0–5.5)	1.4 (.7–1.8)	
Spelling	2.4 (1.2–4.5)	1.9 (.7–3.5)	1.2 (.5–1.8)	
Arithmetic	3.1 (1.9–5.0)	2.4 (1.0–4.5)	1.3 (.3–2.1)	
VADS				VADS Norms
A–O	4.80	4.44	3.94	5.43
V–O	5.19	4.66	3.50	5.91
A–W	4.50	3.88	3.00	5.19
V–W	4.97	4.36	2.72	5.89
A I	9.30	8.34	5.94	10.61
V I	10.13	8.99	6.33	11.80
O E	9.96	9.10	7.44	11.34
W E	9.50	8.25	7.72	11.08
Intra	9.77	8.79	6.66	11.31
Inter	9.70	8.53	6.50	11.10
Total	19.46	17.32	13.17	22.41

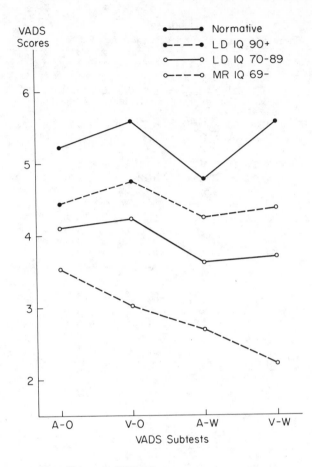

Figure 5. VADS Test mean scores—Age 8.

second-graders in their achievement. Most of the 8- and 9-year-old children
in Group A were able to do some academic work; this was in keeping with
their VADS Test scores. The VADS Test performance of the 8-year-olds was
quite similar to that of average 6½-year-old pupils, whereas the VADS Test
scores of the 9-year-olds were at about the 7-year-old level of the normative
sample.

At age 8 the functioning level of Group B resembled that of beginning
first-grade pupils; by age 9 Group B functioned at the end of first-grade level.

Figure 5 reveals that the VADS Test scores of the 8-year-old LD pupils
in Group A and Group B were beginning to approach the normal VADS Test
score pattern of school-age children. The Visual-Oral and the Visual-Written
Subtest scores were slightly higher than the Aural-Oral and Aural-Written
Subtest Scores. By age 9 the two VADS Subtests with visual input are
markedly higher than the two Subtests with aural input as shown on Figure
6. But even though the test pattern is now normal, the level of all four
Subtests continues to be lower than the level of VADS Test scores of the
average 8- and 9-year-old pupils, just as the achievement level of the LD

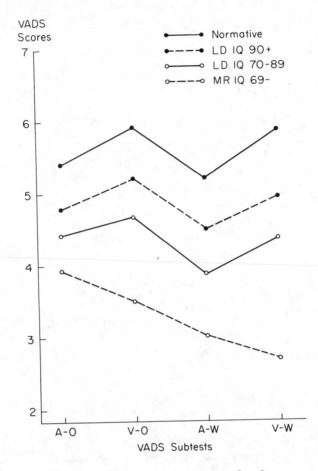

Figure 6. VADS Test mean scores—Age 9.

pupils remains below the expected grade level. The VADS Test mean scores for Group A and Group B are in keeping with the youngsters' achievement scores.

The moderately retarded 8- and 9-year-old children in Group C continued to have some difficulty with the written recall of digits. Their Subtest scores with oral expression (Aural-Oral and Visual-Oral) remain higher than the two Subtest scores with written expression (Aural-Written and Visual-Written). This indicates that the youngsters in Group C had not yet matured in perceptual-motor integration and recall to the level of average 6½-year-old pupils. Academically they were still functioning on the readiness and preprimer level, respectively.

Age 10 and 11

As shown on Table 21 and Table 22, the 10- and 11-year-old LD pupils in Group A were functioning academically on the third- to fourth-grade

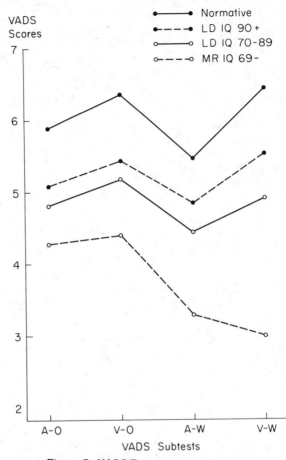

Figure 7. VADS Test mean scores—Age 10.

level; only the spelling scores were consistently lower. Group B was functioning on the second- to third-grade level, and even Group C was beginning to demonstrate first- to second-grade achievement on the Wide Range Achievement Test. The VADS Test scores of Groups A, B, and C all show improvement compared with the 8- and 9-year-old LD pupils.

As can be seen on Figure 7 and Figure 8, by age 10 Group C had slightly higher Visual-Oral than Aural-Oral scores. By age 11 Group C showed for the first time the VADS Subtest score pattern that is typical for average school-age children. The 11-year-old moderately retarded youngsters had gradually matured in perceptual-motor integration and recall to the level where their Visual-Oral and Visual-Written Subtest scores were higher than their Aural-Oral and Aural-Written Subtest scores, although all four Subtest scores were still quite low and resembled those of the 6½-year-old youngsters in the normative sample. Higher scores on the two Subtests with visual input indicate that the pupils were at least able to translate spontaneously visual stimuli into auditory stimuli, and that they used both visual and auditory cues for remembering visually presented digit sequences. Some of the

Table 21.

Characteristics of LD and MR Pupils Age 10–0 to 10–11

	Group A	Group B	Group C	
Age Mean	10–5	10–6	10–4	
Test	Mean (Range)	Mean (Range)	Mean (Range)	
WISC FS IQ	98.3 (90–126)	79.7 (70–89)	61.5 (50–68)	
Bender Test	3.0 (0–13)	5.3 (0–12)	9.1 (4–14)	
WRAT				
Reading Recognition	3.6 (1.4–9.3)	2.7 (1.1–6.1)	2.1 (.7–5.8)	
Spelling	2.9 (1.4–5.3)	2.5 (1.2–5.3)	1.7 (.9–3.5)	
Arithmetic	3.9 (2.1–7.0)	3.1 (1.9–4.7)	1.8 (.6–2.8)	
VADS				VADS Norms
A–O	5.13	4.83	4.30	5.89
V–O	5.46	5.18	4.43	6.34
A–W	4.83	4.47	3.30	5.48
V–W	5.55	4.93	3.00	6.43
A I	9.96	9.30	7.61	11.35
V I	11.01	10.11	7.43	12.77
O E	10.59	10.01	8.73	12.23
W E	10.38	9.40	6.30	11.90
Intra	10.68	9.76	7.30	12.32
Inter	10.29	9.65	7.73	11.82
Total	20.97	19.41	15.03	24.13

Table 22.

Characteristics of LD and MR Pupils Age 11–0 to 11–11

	Group A	Group B	Group C	
Age Mean	11–4	11–5	11–5	
Test	Mean (Range)	Mean (Range)	Mean (Range)	
WISC FS IQ	101.7 (90–128)	78.7 (70–89)	63.0 (54–69)	
Bender Test	2.5 (0–8)	5.1 (0–12)	9.5 (4–15)	
WRAT				
Reading Recognition	4.4 (1.1–9.0)	3.1 (1.1–7.0)	2.5 (1.3–4.8)	
Spelling	3.3 (1.7–6.0)	2.6 (1.4–6.3)	2.1 (1.3–4.8)	
Arithmetic	4.5 (2.8–7.0)	3.4 (1.6–5.3)	1.9 (1.0–3.1)	
VADS				VADS Norms
A–O	5.15	4.74	4.36	5.95
V–O	5.95	5.28	4.64	6.54
A–W	5.24	4.52	4.00	5.74
V–W	5.80	5.20	4.32	6.56
A I	10.39	9.26	8.36	11.69
V I	11.75	10.48	8.96	13.10
O E	11.10	10.02	9.00	12.49
W E	11.04	9.72	8.32	12.30
Intra	10.95	9.94	8.68	12.51
Inter	11.19	9.80	8.64	12.28
Total	22.14	19.74	17.32	24.79

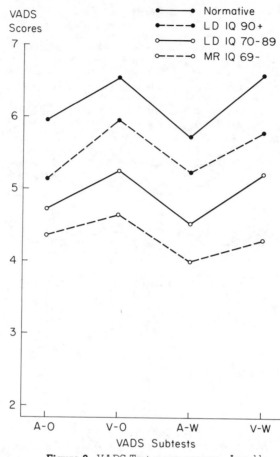

Figure 8. VADS Test mean scores—Age 11.

youngsters had also learned to group or chunk the digits to facilitate their recall.

Although all three groups of LD and MR youngsters continued to improve on the VADS Test scores from age 5½ to 11 years, none of them had been able to "catch up" with the VADS Test performance of average school-children at any given age level. The latter also kept improving on their VADS Test performances. In fact, the discrepancy between the VADS Test scores of the LD pupils and of the normative sample increased as the youngsters got older. At age 8, the Total VADS Test scores of the LD pupils in Group A lagged only 1½ years behind the Total VADS Test scores of the normative sample; they resembled the scores of average 6½-year-olds. At age 10, the Total VADS Test scores of the children in Group A resembled those of average 8-year-olds, that is, they lagged 2 years behind the Total VADS Test scores of normal 10-year-old pupils.

Age 12 to 14

Table 23 reveals that the 12-year-old LD pupils in Group A progressed

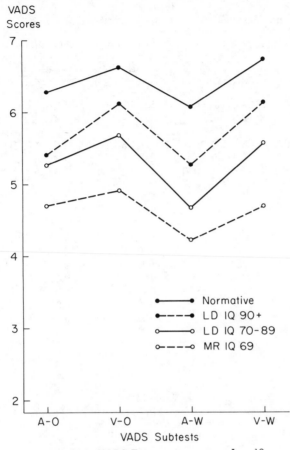

Figure 9. VADS Test mean scores—Age 12.

in reading recognition and arithmetic to the end-of-fourth to beginning-fifth grade level; only their spelling scores remained on the third-grade level. The 12-year-old youngsters in Group B were found to function on the third-grade level, whereas the moderately retarded pupils in Group C had an average second-grade achievement. All three groups showed a marked improvement, between the ages of 11 and 12, on their achievement and VADS Test scores. But, as before, there was still a large discrepancy between the achievement and VADS Test scores of Group A and Group B, between the scores of Group B and Group C, and between all three groups and the normative sample of 12-year-old pupils. Figure 9 shows these discrepancies graphically.

The achievement and the VADS Test score means for 13- and 14-year-old LD and MR pupils, as presented on Table 24, showed a very different picture from that of the 12-year-old LD and MR pupils. Until age 12 there had been from year to year a steady increase in Group A on the achievement and VADS Test scores. By age 13 and 14, the LD pupils with average mental potential, who were still in need of special education, seemed to reach a plateau and failed to show any improvement on their achievement and VADS Test scores.

Table 23.

Characteristics of LD and MR Pupils Age 12–0 to 12–11

	Group A	Group B	Group C	
Age Mean	12–4	12–5	12–5	
Test	Mean (Range)	Mean (Range)	Mean (Range)	
WISC FS IQ	99.6 (90–118)	78.2 (70–89)	60.9 (48–69)	
Bender Test	2.3 (0–7)	4.4 (0–12)	8.4 (4–20)	
WRAT				
Reading Recognition	5.1 (2.0–12.0)	3.6 (1.5–7.8)	3.0 (1.1–6.7)	
Spelling	3.8 (2.0–8.7)	3.0 (1.5–5.5)	2.3 (1.2–6.5)	
Arithmetic	5.1 (3.2–10.7)	4.0 (2.4–5.9)	2.5 (1.6–3.9)	
VADS				VADS Norms
A–O	5.43	5.29	4.69	6.27
V–O	6.11	5.68	4.94	6.62
A–W	5.27	4.66	4.25	6.09
V–W	6.14	5.61	4.69	6.69
A I	10.70	9.95	8.94	12.36
V I	12.25	11.29	9.63	13.31
O E	11.54	10.97	9.63	12.89
W E	11.41	10.27	8.94	12.78
Intra	11.57	10.90	9.38	12.96
Inter	11.38	10.34	9.19	12.71
Total	22.95	21.24	18.57	25.67

Table 24.

Characteristics of LD and MR Pupils Age 13–0 to 14–11

	Group A	Group B	Group C	
Age Mean	13–7	13–10	13–9	
Test	Mean (Range)	Mean (Range)	Mean (Range)	
WISC FS IQ	97.8 (90–124)	80.1 (70–89)	62.1 (52–69)	
Bender Test	1.4 (0–6)	3.1 (0–8)	6.2 (1–17)	
WRAT				
Reading Recognition	4.8 (1.6–10.8)	4.5 (2.0–11.5)	3.4 (.9–7.2)	
Spelling	3.7 (1.7–9.2)	3.6 (1.8–6.5)	3.2 (1.2–7.7)	
Arithmetic	4.9 (2.9–10.0)	4.5 (2.8–7.0)	3.4 (1.9–6.1)	
VADS				VADS Norms (CA 12)
A–O	5.50	5.42	4.54	6.27
V–O	6.03	6.08	5.61	6.62
A–W	5.18	5.21	4.38	6.09
V–W	6.05	5.96	5.38	6.69
A I	10.68	10.63	8.92	12.36
V I	12.08	12.04	10.99	13.31
O E	11.53	11.50	10.15	12.89
W E	11.23	11.17	9.76	12.78
Intra	11.55	11.38	9.92	12.96
Inter	11.21	11.29	9.99	12.71
Total	22.76	22.67	19.91	25.67

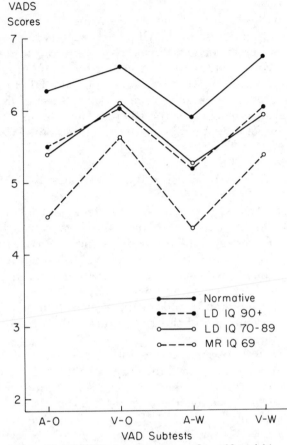

VADS
Scores

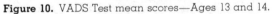

Figure 10. VADS Test mean scores—Ages 13 and 14.

By contrast, the 13- and 14-year-old children of dull normal to borderline mental ability in Group B continued to show progress in both achievement and VADS Test performance. In fact, they actually caught up with the level of achievement and the VADS Test scores of the brighter 13- and 14-year-old LD pupils in Group A. As can be seen on Figure 10, the VADS Test performance of Group A and Group B was almost identical.

At age 13 and 14, the moderately retarded youngsters in Group C functioned academically at the beginning third-grade level and they showed ongoing improvement on their VADS Test scores. Their VADS Test score means resembled those of normal 7-year-old pupils.

Thus, it appears that in Group B and Group C, the youngsters with more limited mental ability continue to progress in their achievement and on the VADS Test at least up to age 14, whereas the brighter youngsters with severe learning disabilities in Group A, as a group, failed to show any improvement in their achievement and on the VADS Test after age 12. This global picture refers, of course, to a whole group of youngsters with normal mental ability who had very serious learning difficulties and who were still in need of special education. However, within this group there were individual differences between the children. Some of the 13- and 14-year-old pupils in Group A did continue to progress in their functioning level beyond age 12. More longitudinal and cross-sectional research is required to determine at what point the low average and borderline youngsters in Group B and the moderately retarded pupils in Group C level off and fail to show any more significant progress in their achievement and in the VADS Test scores, and whether the plateau reached by the LD pupils in Group A is only temporary or whether they continue to improve in their functioning level after puberty.

LD AND MR PUPILS AGE 6½ TO 14: SUMMARY

The VADS Test score means and achievement levels of LD and MR pupils, age 6½ to 14 years, were compared with each other and with the VADS Test performance of the normative sample. Up to age 12, the findings were quite consistent: the VADS Test scores of LD and MR pupils follow the same developmental sequence as those of average public school students, only at a much slower rate. Figure 11 compares the rate of maturation in perceptual-motor integration and recall, as measured on the VADS Test, of the normative sample and of the LD pupils with normal mental ability in Group A at different age levels.

The similarity between the developmental stages of the two groups is striking. As shown on Figure 11, the 6½-year-old LD pupils had VADS Test scores that were very much like those of average kindergarten youngsters age 5½; this means that the 6½-year-old LD pupils lagged about 1 year behind average pupils on their VADS Test performance. By age 8, the VADS Test scores of the LD pupils had progressed to the level of 6½-year-old normal children. Therefore, the 8-year-old LD youngsters lagged 1½ years behind the normative sample in their development in perceptual-motor integration and recall.

By age 10, the VADS Test performance of the LD pupils was almost identical with that of average 8-year-old youngsters; so that a 2-year lag had developed between the VADS Test scores of the LD youngsters and normal pupils age 10. This discrepancy increased to 2½ years by age 12. The VADS Test scores of 12-year-old LD pupils fell between those of the 9- and 10-year-old pupils of the normative sample. After age 12, at ages 13 and 14, the VADS Test scores of the LD pupils of average mental ability no longer improved. Thus, it appears that the VADS Test scores of LD pupils not only fail to catch up with the VADS Test scores of average pupils but they actually fall farther behind as the youngsters get older. These findings are significant since so many LD pupils, despite their average mental ability, reach a plateau in their schoolwork and fail to progress academically beyond the end-of-fourth or beginning fifth-grade level. The relationship between the VADS Test scores and the achievement level of the LD pupils is striking. The question that presents itself is whether the LD pupils could improve their achievement if they could improve their ability in perceptual-motor integration, sequencing, and recall. Has enough effort been made to teach children how to

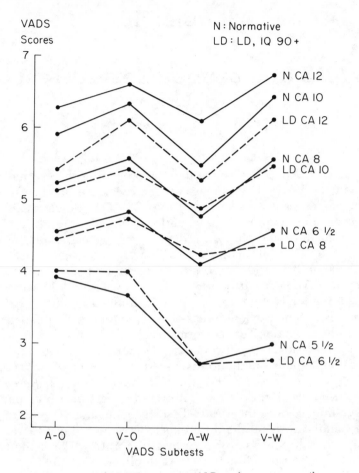

Figure 11. VADS Test scores of LD and average pupils.

organize and remember information so they can recall it later on? How well can integration and memory be taught or are they mainly related to maturation and neurological functioning?

Dull normal and borderline youngsters with learning difficulties progressed in their achievement and VADS Test performance at a slower rate than LD pupils of average mental ability. However, by age 13 and 14, the functioning level of the slower children had continued to improve and had caught up with the VADS Test performance of the brighter LD pupils. Moderately retarded youngsters' achievement and progress on the VADS Test improved at an even slower rate than that of the dull normal pupils.

More research is needed to discover how long and how far the slower LD and MR pupils are able to improve their achievement and VADS Test performance, and whether the plateau in achievement and VADS Test performance, reached by the brighter LD pupils at age 12, is only a temporary one or whether it is permanent.

Chapter 10

The VADS and Bender Gestalt Test of LD Pupils

Many of the LD pupils, discussed in the preceding chapter, had not only difficulty with the VADS Test but also did poorly on the Bender Gestalt Test (Bender, 1938) as can be seen on Table 25. The Bender Gestalt Test performances of both Group A (IQ 90 and above) and Group B (IQ 70 to 89) were quite immature and showed a developmental lag similar to the one displayed by the LD pupils on the VADS Test. The 6½-year-old LD pupils of average mental ability produced Bender Gestalt Test scores that were like those of normal 5½-year-old children. The 10-year-old LD youngsters in Group A had Bender Test scores that were similar to the scores of average 8-year-old pupils, whereas the 11-year-old LD pupils resembled normal 9-year-olds on their Bender Test performance.

The close relationship between the Bender Gestalt Test and learning difficulties was demonstrated and discussed at great length in *The Bender Gestalt Test for young children, Volume I* and *Volume II, Research and application* (Koppitz, 1963, 1975a). The Bender Test measures perceptual-motor integration, as does the VADS Test. It seems therefore appropriate to explore the similarities and the differences between the two tests and their relationship to each other and to learning disabilities. For if the two tests measure mainly the same functions and duplicate each other, then there would be little justification for using both tests when diagnosing learning problems in school children.

The standardized administration of the Bender Test requires that a youngster copy nine moderately complex, abstract designs from stimulus cards that remain on the table in full view until the drawings have been completed. In order to do well on the Bender Test a child has to be able to perceive and analyze visual configurations in terms of their details, relative size, direction, and spatial relationships, and he has to reproduce the designs, as accurately as possible, with a pencil on paper. Thus, the Bender Gestalt Test involves visual perception, visual analysis, the understanding of part-whole relationships, and the integration of all of these with grapho-motor expression. The Standard Bender Gestalt Test does not involve language skills, nor does it depend on the ability to sequence and recall the designs; it has also no time limits.

The VADS Test differs greatly from the Bender Test in that it uses series of familiar digits as stimuli; furthermore these are presented for only a brief period of time, and the youngsters have to reproduce them in the exact sequence from memory. The VADS Test involves visual as well as auditory

Table 25.
Bender Test Mean Scores of LD and Average Pupils

Age	Group A LD (IQ 90 +) Mean (Range)	Group B LD (IQ 70–89) Mean (Range)	Normative[1]
5–6/5–11	—	—	9.7[2]
6–0/6–5	—	—	8.6
6–6/6–11	9.6 (4–13)	12.4 (7–16)	7.2
7–0/7–11	7.5 (1–14)	10.1 (1–15)	4.8
8–0/8–11	5.5 (0–12)	9.1 (4–17)	3.1
9–0/9–11	3.9 (0–12)	6.8 (1–14)	2.1
10–0/10–11	3.0 (0–13)	5.3 (0–12)	1.5
11–0/11–11	2.5 (0–8)	5.1 (0–12)	1.4
12–0/12–11	2.3 (0–7)	4.4 (0–12)	—
13–0/14–11	1.4 (0–6)	3.1 (0–8)	—

[1]The Bender Test normative data were derived from Tables 4 and 5 of *The Bender Gestalt Test for young children, Volume II, Research and application, 1963–1973* (Koppitz, 1975a).

[2]A high Bender Test score is a poor score since the test is scored for imperfections.

perception, integration, and recall. The VADS Test is more difficult than the Bender Test since it requires not only visual-motor integration but also auditory-visual and visual-oral integration and sequencing and recall. The Bender Test is mainly a test of visual analysis and visual-motor perception.

The Bender Test Recall method (Koppitz, 1975a, p. 120) is a modification of the standard Bender Test. It assesses youngsters' ability to draw the Bender Test designs from memory. This memory task is quite different from the memory task on the VADS Test. The Bender Test Recall is not concerned with the recall of specific symbol sequences in different sense modalities. The Bender Test does not involve language, and the designs have little resemblance to the symbols, letters, and digits used in writing and reading. Hence, it is not surprising that research with the Bender Test Recall method failed to show a close relationship between it and reading achievement.

In an earlier study (Koppitz, 1973), I compared the VADS Test and the Bender Gestalt Test performance of 30 learning-disabled boys, age 9 and 10 years, (IQ mean 90, IQ range 71 to 106) with those of 20 normal school-children who had the same age, mental ability, and socioeconomic background. Significant differences were obtained, when using the Chi-square statistic, between the LD youngsters and the control group on the Bender Test and on three of the four VADS Subtest scores and the Total VADS Test score. Only the Aural-Oral Subtest failed to differentiate between the two groups of boys. Thus, it appears that both the VADS Test and the Bender Test can distinguish between children with and without learning problems.

In another study (Koppitz, 1975b), I explored the differences between the VADS Test and the Bender Gestalt Test scores of two groups of 8- and 9-year-old LD pupils of average mental ability (IQ 90 to 118) and a matched control group. One of the LD groups was made up of nonreaders, whereas the other LD group had only moderate reading problems but showed serious emotional and behavior difficulties. The VADS Test was able to discriminate between the readers and nonreaders among the LD pupils; the Bender Gestalt Test was unable to do so. On the other hand, the VADS Test could only differentiate between the LD youngsters who could not read and the control group, but not between the LD pupils with moderate reading problems and the controls. The Bender Test could not distinguish between the two LD groups, but it was able to discriminate both groups of LD youngsters from the normal pupils.

No statistically significant relationships were found between the VADS Test scores and the Bender Test scores of the two LD groups or of the control group. The results of this study suggest that the VADS Test and the Bender Gestalt Test are both related to learning disabilities but they are independent of each other. The Bender Test is more closely related to overall school functioning than to reading achievement in particular, whereas the VADS Test is specifically related to achievement but not to children's overall school adjustment and functioning.

In order to explore the relationship of all 11 VADS Test measures with the Bender Gestalt Test scores of younger and older children and of youngsters of average and of below average mental ability, I correlated the VADS Test and Bender Test scores of 193 LD pupils. These pupils included all 8- and 10-year-olds from the LD sample (Table 16) to whom I had administered the VADS Test and the Bender Test at the same session. Both the 8- and 10-year-old children were divided into two groups; one group included only children with at least average mental ability (WISC FS IQ 90 or above), the other group consisted of youngsters of low average to borderline mental ability (WISC FS IQ 70 to 89). Thus, the VADS Test and the Bender Test scores came from the following four groups of LD pupils:

Group I: N 51, Age 8, IQ 70 to 89;
Group II: N 50, Age 8, IQ 90 or above;
Group III: N 47, Age 10, IQ 70 to 89;
Group IV: N 45, Age 10, IQ 90 or above.

Of the 44 correlations computed for the 11 VADS Test measures and the Bender Test scores of the four groups, only five were statistically significant.

Group I: Four of the 11 VADS Test measures were found to be related to the Bender Test Scores of 8-year-old LD pupils with below average mental ability. These four VADS Test measures were the Visual-Written Subtest ($r = -.29$,[1] $p < .05$), Visual Input ($r = -.32$, $p < .05$), Written Expression ($r = -.29$, p < .05), and Intersensory Integration ($r = -.32$, p < .05). It appears that younger and duller children, with as yet immature visual-motor perception and lack of recall strategies, have difficulties on both

---

[1]Since the VADS Test is scored for achievement and the Bender Test is scored for errors, a positive correlation between the two sets of scores results in a negative coefficient.

the Bender Gestalt Test and the VADS Test measures that involve visual-motor integration.

Group II: For 8-year-old LD children of normal mental ability only the Visual-Written Subtest scores were significantly related to the Bender Test scores ($r = -.27$, p $<$ .05). Both tests involve primarily visual-motor perception. None of the other VADS Test measures was significantly related to the Bender Test scores of the 8-year-old LD pupils with average IQ scores.

Group III and IV: None of the 11 VADS Test measures was found to be significantly related to the Bender Gestalt Test scores of the 10-year-old LD pupils of average and of below average mental ability. Since many of the 10-year-old youngsters use verbal rehearsal when recalling the visually presented digits on the Visual-Written Subtest, this VADS Subtest ceases to be exclusively a test of visual-motor perception for all children. In consequence, the Visual-Written Subtest was no longer significantly related to the Bender Test scores of the 10-year-old LD pupils. Both the Bender Test and the VADS Test are associated with learning problems, but apparently they measure different aspects of such difficulties and supplement each other.

We examine next how often LD pupils, age 7 to 14, exhibit poor scores on both the VADS Test and the Bender Test, or whether youngsters with learning disabilities are more apt to have difficulties with one or the other of the two tests. The Bender Test and VADS Test scores of the LD pupils were divided into "average" and "low" or "poor" scores. An "average" score was defined as being less than minus one standard deviation from the mean score for a given age level. A "low" or "poor" VADS Test or Bender Test score was defined as being at or more than one standard deviation from the mean score for a given age level. The means and standard deviations for the VADS Test were taken from Table 7 (p. 62), and the means and standard deviations for the Bender Gestalt Test were found on Table 5 and Table 11 of *The Bender Gestalt Test for young children, Volume II, Research and application, 1963–1973* (Koppitz, 1975a).

Table 26 shows the percentage of 302 LD pupils of average mental ability (IQ 90 or above) with poor VADS Test and Bender Test scores. It can be seen that 74% of the 7-year-old LD pupils had very low VADS Test scores, as did 59 to 70% of the LD youngsters age 8 to 14. The proportion of LD children who had poor Bender Test scores was considerably smaller. Of the 7- and 8-year-old LD children 45% had very low Bender Test scores; the same was true for 33 to 37% of the 9- to 12-year-old pupils, and for 17% of the 13- and 14-year-old LD students.

It should be noted that the ceiling of the Bender Test is lower than the ceiling of the VADS Test. The VADS Test is the more difficult of the two tests. Many LD pupils, age 10 to 14, are able to complete the Bender Gestalt Test with few if any errors, while they continue to have difficulties with the VADS Test. Therefore, the percentage of LD pupils with poor Bender Test scores decreases more rapidly, as the children get older, than the percentage of LD youngsters with poor VADS Test scores. The VADS Test is therefore of particular value for the older LD pupils.

Table 26.

Percentage of LD Pupils (IQ 90 and above) With Poor VADS and Bender Test Scores

Test	Age 7 (N 31)	Age 8 (N 49)	Age 9 (N 65)	Age 10 (N 51)	Age 11 (N 40)	Age 12 (N 36)	Age 13 & 14 (N 30)
Poor VADS[1]	74%	64%	59%	59%	63%	70%	70%
Poor Bender	45%	45%	37%	36%	33%	36%	17%
Average VADS[2]	16%	22%	20%	23%	32%	25%	23%
Average Bender							
Average VADS	10%	14%	21%	18%	5%	5%	7%
Poor Bender							
Poor VADS	39%	33%	43%	41%	35%	39%	60%
Average Bender							
Poor VADS	35%	31%	16%	18%	28%	31%	10%
Poor Bender							

[1] A "Poor" score is defined as being minus one standard deviation or more from the mean VADS Test or Bender Test score for a given age level.

[2] An "Average" score is defined as being less than minus one standard deviation from the mean VADS Test or Bender Test score for a given age level.

When the VADS Test and the Bender Test scores were considered together, it was found that from 20 to 32% of the 8- to 14-year-old LD children scored in the average range on both of the tests, but only 16% of the 7-year-old pupils did likewise. However, a test score that is close to the lower border of the average range is still a weak score. The case of John serves to illustrate this point. John, age 8 years 11 months, had a Total VADS Test score of 19 and a Bender Test score of 5; both scores were just within the normal range. An analysis of John's VADS Test scores showed that his visual recall was good; he had a Visual Input score of 12. His auditory processing on the other hand was very poor; his Aural Input score was only 7. Even though the Total VADS Test score was low average, the VADS Subtests revealed that John had a specific language problem. Language difficulties were also shown by the discrepancy between John's WISC Verbal IQ score of 106 and his Performance IQ score of 120. His Full Scale IQ score was 114. In view of John's superior Performance IQ score, his low average score of 5 on the Bender Gestalt Test had to be regarded as unusually poor. It is characteristic of LD pupils of normal intelligence that their Bender Test scores are considerably lower than their mental age warrants (Koppitz, 1975a, p. 81). A meaningful assessment of both the VADS Test and the Bender Test scores can only be made when the child's age and mental ability are taken into account, and when not only the Total VADS Test score but also the various VADS Subtests and Combination scores are analyzed in relation to each other.

Table 26 shows that between 5 and 21% of the LD pupils had VADS Test scores that were in the average range, whereas their Bender Test scores were very poor. Thus, LD children may do poorly on only one of the two tests. The Bender Gestalt Test seems to be able to identify some youngsters with problems that the VADS Test cannot identify. An example of such a situation was demonstrated by Jeff's test performance. Jeff, age 11 years, was a bright, verbal youngster with a WISC Verbal IQ of 111, a Performance IQ of 105, and a Full Scale IQ of 109. His VADS Test score of 24 was within the normal range. He showed no serious difficulty with the sequencing and recall of digit sequences. Jeff was one of those verbal, impulsive, disorganized, hyperactive, poorly coordinated, and poorly controlled children with a low frustration tolerance and immature visual-motor perception who fail in school despite good mental ability. His reasoning was good but he could not settle down and concentrate. Jeff disrupted other children and rarely completed his assignments. His Bender Test record was extremely disorganized and immature; it reflected his actual level of functioning in school. The Bender Test score of 5 was on the level of 7-year-old children.

Table 26 reveals that between 33% and 43% of the LD youngsters, age 7 to 12, obtained very low scores on the VADS Test, whereas their Bender Test scores were in the normal range, and as many as 60% of the 13- and 14-year-old LD pupils had poor VADS Test scores even though their Bender Test scores were at least average. It appears, therefore, that the VADS Test alone can identify a larger number of LD pupils than the Bender Test by itself. Because of its low ceiling, the Bender Test could no longer differen-

tiate effectively between 13- and 14-year-old pupils with and without learning problems (Koppitz, 1975a, p. 13). This was well illustrated by the case of
Warren, age 13 years 5 months.

Warren's Bender Test score of 1 was quite good, whereas, his Total
VADS Test score of 17 was very poor. His near perfect Bender Test performance merely indicated that, at age 13½, Warren's visual-motor perception
was on the level of normal 10-year-old children, who can also produce near
perfect Bender Test records. Once a Bender Test score is perfect or near
perfect it cannot improve any more, and the Bender Test can no longer
distinguish between average and above average performances.

Warren learned best from material he could see and manipulate and he
also liked to draw. His language skills and abstract reasoning were very
limited, and his memory for sounds and symbols was poor. He obtained a
WISC Verbal IQ of 85, a Performance IQ of 103, and a Full Scale IQ of 93.
The low Verbal IQ score, especially the low scores on Information (long-
term memory for facts and figures), Arithmetic (auditory processing and
recall), and Digit Span (sequencing and short-term memory), are in keeping
with Warren's poor VADS Test, and are characteristic of children with severe
learning problems (Koppitz, 1971, p. 121). Warren's reading and writing
were only on the second- to third-grade level.

From 16% to 35% of the 7- to 12-year-old LD pupils with average mental
ability revealed poor scores on both the VADS Test *and* the Bender Test
(Table 26); so did 10% of the 13- and 14-year-olds. As was shown previously,
most of the older LD pupils were able to produce relatively good Bender
Test records; only the VADS Test continued to discriminate between LD
and normal pupils up to age 14.

If a child displays either a very poor Bender Test score *or* a very low
VADS Test score he may also have learning difficulties; but when a youngster shows a poor performance on both the Bender Test *and* the VADS Test
then the presence of learning problems is almost certain. Tammy is a good
example of such a pupil. Tammy was an outgoing, bright girl of 7½ years,
who was a nonreader despite a WISC Verbal IQ of 111, a Performance IQ of
104, and a Full Scale IQ of 107. Tammy had very immature visual-motor
perception and a severe memory deficit for sound and symbol association.
Her Bender Test score of 14 was still on the preschool level, whereas her
VADS Test score of 13 resembled that of a 5-year-old child. Tammy was as
yet on the readiness level in reading and writing even though she had
received individual tutoring at home and special help in school.

So far we have only considered LD pupils of average mental ability.
Now we examine the occurrence of poor VADS Test and Bender Test scores
among children with learning problems who have only dull average or
borderline mental ability. Table 27 shows the percentage of 7- to 14-year-old
slow LD pupils (IQ 70 to 89) who had poor VADS Test and poor Bender Test
scores. It can be seen that the duller youngsters had a much higher incidence
of poor scores on both the VADS Test and the Bender Test than did the LD
pupils of average intelligence. As many as 91% of the 7-year-old and 85% of
the 8-year-old slow LD pupils showed extremely low VADS Test scores, as

Table 27.

Percentage of LD Pupils (QI 70–89) With Poor VADS and Bender Test Scores

Test	Age 7 (N 24)	Age 8 (N 60)	Age 9 (N 65)	Age 10 (N 68)	Age 11 (N 51)	Age 12 (N 39)	Age 13 & 14 (N 42)
Poor VADS[1]	91%	85%	76%	75%	79%	77%	74%
Poor Bender	66%	81%	72%	71%	87%	77%	62%
Average VADS[2] } Average Bender	0%	7%	6%	7%	4%	8%	9%
Average VADS } Poor Bender	8%	8%	18%	18%	18%	15%	17%
Poor VADS } Average Bender	33%	12%	22%	22%	10%	15%	29%
Poor VADS } Poor Bender	58%	73%	54%	53%	69%	62%	45%

[1] A "Poor" score is defined as being minus one standard deviation or more from the mean VADS Test or Bender Test score for a given age level.
[2] An "Average" score is defined as being less than minus one standard deviation from the mean VADS Test or Bender Test score for a given age level.

did 74 to 79% of the 9- to 14-year-old youngsters. The percentage of dull normal to borderline LD pupils with poor Bender Test scores ranged from a low of 62%, for 13- and 14-year-olds, to a high of 87%, for 11-year-olds.

When the VADS Test and the Bender Test were considered together, it was found that none of the 7-year-old duller LD pupils scored within the average range on both of the tests. Of the LD pupils age 8 to 11, only 4 to 7% did relatively well on both the VADS and the Bender Test, whereas 8 to 9% of the 12- to 14-year-olds scored within the normal range on the VADS Test as well as on the Bender Test.

Of the 7- and 8-year-old slow LD pupils 8% displayed relatively high VADS Test scores along with very poor Bender Test scores. For the older LD pupils, age 9 to 14 years, 15 to 18% fell into this category. A somewhat larger percentage of the slow LD pupils showed poor VADS Test scores together with relatively good Bender Test scores, whereas 45 to 73% of the dull normal and borderline LD youngsters, age 7 to 14, scored poorly on both the VADS Test and the Bender Test.

The results on Table 27 suggest that the majority of slow pupils with serious learning problems had very poor perceptual-motor integration and recall. As shown previously, the presence of either a very poor Bender Test score or a very low VADS Test score can reflect specific learning difficulties; but when a child, age 7 to 11, obtains poor scores on both the VADS Test and the Bender Test, then he is almost certain to have serious learning disabilities. However, even when a child has relatively good scores on both the VADS Test and the Bender Test, learning difficulties cannot be entirely ruled out, especially for pupils age 12 to 14. A case in point was Charlie.

Charlie, age 14 years, 8 months, had good short-term memory and recall; his VADS Test scores were excellent. He obtained an Aural-Oral score of 7, a Visual-Oral score of 7, an Aural-Written score of 6, and a Visual-Written score of 7, with a Total VADS Test score of 27. He also had no difficulty copying the nine Bender Test designs without error, a minor irregularity on the Bender Test record resulted in a score of 1. Charlie's VADS Test and Bender Test performances were on the level of 11- and 12-year-old children; by contrast, his school achievement was quite poor. Charlie's reading recognition and decoding skill was fair as a result of his good recall, but his reading comprehension was extremely low (fourth-grade level), as was his understanding of number concepts. Charlie was a dull youngster who learned mainly by rote. His WISC Verbal IQ was 86, his Performance IQ was 78, and his Full Scale IQ was 80. Charlie had poor language skills and dropped word endings when he spoke or wrote; in addition, he was turned off by school and was grossly lacking in motivation for schoolwork. As soon as he turned 16, Charlie dropped out of school and went to work. In Charlie's case neither the VADS Test nor the Bender Test was able to diagnose his poor achievement since he was not a youngster with specific learning disabilities. Charlie's low achievement was the result of social and emotional deprivation and of poor reasoning ability. None of this is reflected on the VADS Test scores or on the Bender Test scores of older pupils.

THE VADS AND BENDER TEST OF LD PUPILS: SUMMARY

Research revealed that both the VADS Test and the Bender Test are related to learning disabilities, but the Bender Test is more closely associated with overall school functioning whereas the VADS Test is more closely related to reading, spelling, and arithmetic achievement. The two tests are independent of each other; they measure different aspects of learning problems and supplement each other.

The Bender Test is the easier one to master of the two tests; therefore, it identifies learning problems less well among older pupils than the VADS Test. Among LD children of average mental ability half of the younger children had poor Bender Test scores, but by age 9 to 12 only one-third of the youngsters did poorly on the Bender Test; on the VADS Test roughly three-fourths to two-thirds of the LD pupils at all age levels, 7 to 14 years, produced poor scores. Among low average and borderline pupils with learning problems, age 7 to 14, the incidence of poor test scores was much higher for both tests. In ranged from 91 to 74% for the VADS Test, and from 81 to 62% for the Bender Test. A given LD pupil may obtain either a very low VADS Test score or a very poor Bender Test score, or both. The presence of either one or two poor scores on these tests is diagnostically highly significant.

Chapter 11

VADS Test and Achievement of LD Pupils

As was shown previously, the VADS Test scores are related to the achievement of public school children, and they can discriminate between groups of average and learning-disabled pupils. In this chapter, we explore in detail the relationship of VADS Test scores and the achievement of groups of pupils with learning disabilities. The subjects for this study were 104 8-year-old and 92 10-year-old youngsters from the LD sample to whom I had administered the VADS Test and the complete Wide Range Achievement Test at the same testing session. The 196 children were divided into four groups according to their age and WISC Full Scale IQ scores. The age, IQ, and achievement levels of the four groups are shown on Table 28.

The 11 VADS Test measures were correlated with the Wide Range Achievement Test Reading Recognition, Spelling, and Arithmetic scores for each of the four groups of LD pupils. The results are presented on Table 29. Of the 132 correlation coefficients obtained, all but 11 were statistically significant; 14 were significant at the .05 level, and 107 were significant at the .01 level or better. It is apparent that the VADS Test performance of the four groups of LD pupils was closely related to their level of achievement with one exception. This one exception was the Aural-Oral Subtest.

The Aural-Oral Subtest failed to show significant correlations with any of the three achievement measures for the duller 8-year-olds and the brighter 10-year-olds (Group I and IV), and for the arithmetic scores of the brighter 8-year-olds (Group II). Of the remaining correlations with the Aural-Oral Subtest four were significant at the .05 level and only one (Spelling for the duller 10-year-olds in Group III) reached the .01 level. With a few minor exceptions, all the correlations between the other 10 VADS Test measures and the achievement scores were statistically highly significant.

For Group I (duller 8-year-old LD) the highest correlation coefficients were found for the Reading Recognition and Spelling scores and the Visual-Oral, Visual Input, and Intersensory Integration scores on the VADS. However, all other VADS Test measures, with the exception of the Aural-Oral Subtest, were also associated with reading recognition and spelling achievement. The Arithmetic scores correlated most highly with the Visual-Oral, Visual-Written, Written Expression, Intrasensory and Intersensory Integration, and with the Total VADS Test scores. Arithmetic scores were not significantly related to the Aural-Oral and Aural-Written Subtest scores. That is, for younger, immature children with learning problems, visual-motor integration and visual memory were more closely associated with arithmetic than were auditory processing and recall.

For Group II (brighter 8-year-old LDs), the Reading and Spelling scores correlated significantly with all 11 VADS Test measures, but the correlations

Table 28.
Four Groups of Learning-Disabled Pupils

Test	Group I CA 8 (N 54) Mean (Range)	Group II CA 8 (N 50) Mean (Range)	Group III CA 10 (N 47) Mean (Range)	Group IV CA 10 (N 45) Mean (Range)
WISC FS IQ	81.6 (70–89)	101.3 (90–127)	78.4 (70–89)	98.6 (90–113)
WRAT				
Reading Recognition	1.6 (.2–4.4)	2.5 (1.1–7.0)	2.6 (1.0–6.1)	3.5 (1.4–9.3)
Spelling	1.5 (.1–2.9)	2.1 (.8–4.7)	2.4 (1.2–5.3)	2.9 (1.4–5.3)
Arithmetic	1.8 (.3–3.0)	2.7 (1.5–4.5)	3.0 (1.9–4.7)	3.5 (2.1–5.7)

between Aural-Oral and Aural-Written scores and reading and spelling were somewhat lower (p < .05) than the other nine correlations (p < .01). The Arithmetic scores correlated best with the Visual-Oral, Visual-Written, Visual Input, Oral Expression, Intersensory Integration, and the Total VADS Test scores. Once again, the Aural-Oral and the Aural-Written Subtests were not associated with Arithmetic achievement.

Group III (duller 10-year-old LDs) showed the highest correlations of the four groups of LD pupils between achievement scores, as measured on the Wide Range Achievement Test, and the VADS Test performance. All 33 correlations, between the 11 VADS Test measures and the Reading, Spelling, and Arithmetic scores, were statistically significant. The relatively lowest correlations occurred with the Aural-Oral and Aural-Written Subests, but even these were significant at the .05 and .01 level. The association between Reading Recognition and Spelling and the VADS Test was somewhat closer than with the Arithmetic scores, but this difference was insignificant.

For Group IV (brighter 10-year-old LDs) the achievement scores correlated significantly with all VADS Test measures but the Aural-Oral Subtest. Reading, Spelling, and Arithmetic were most closely associated with the Visual-Oral, Visual Input, Written Expression, Intersensory Integration and the Total VADS Test scores.

Considered as a whole, the findings on Table 29 show that all the VADS Test measures, with the possible exception of the Aural-Oral Subtest, are closely related to the achievement of children with learning disabilities.

Among the duller LD children (IQ 70 to 89) the association between achievement scores and the VADS Test performance was closer for the older (CA 10) than for the younger (CA 8) pupils. For LD youngsters of average mental ability (IQ 90 or above) the correlations between the achievement and the VADS Test measures were somewhat higher for the younger (CA 8) than for the older (CA 10) group of LD pupils. The relationship between the achievement and VADS Test scores was significantly closer for all four groups of LD children than for the normal fifth-grade students discussed previously.

The foregoing study was conducted to demonstrate the validity of the VADS Test as a diagnostic instrument for problems in reading recognition, spelling, and arithmetic. However, the close correlation between the VADS

Table 29.

Correlations between VADS and Wide Range Achievement Test Scores of LD Pupils

VADS	Group I			Group II			Group III			Group IV		
	Reading	Spelling	Arithmetic	Reading	Spelling	Arithmetic	Reading	Spelling	Arithmetic	Reading	Spelling	Arithmetic
A–O	.17	.12	.09	.35*	.29*	.13	.33*	.41**	.34*	.10	.04	.23
V–O	.44**	.43**	.45**	.50**	.58**	.56**	.59**	.50**	.47**	.55**	.53**	.55**
A–W	.39**	.31*	.17	.34*	.39**	.14	.47**	.48**	.38**	.42**	.35*	.44**
V–W	.31*	.38**	.60**	.54**	.59**	.51**	.50**	.47**	.52**	.43**	.39**	.49**
A I	.39**	.27	.33*	.38**	.38**	.15	.50**	.54**	.40**	.32*	.27	.40**
V I	.42**	.46**	.35**	.57**	.64**	.59**	.61**	.54**	.56**	.57**	.54**	.61**
O E	.44**	.35**	.37**	.51**	.53**	.48**	.60**	.59**	.53**	.42**	.39**	.48**
W E	.38**	.38**	.57**	.51**	.57**	.39**	.60**	.63**	.50**	.49**	.43**	.54**
Intra	.36**	.35**	.50**	.52**	.53**	.39**	.51**	.53**	.53**	.35*	.30*	.48**
Inter	.68**	.61**	.73**	.51**	.59**	.43**	.65**	.64**	.52**	.54**	.50**	.56**
Total	.29*	.42**	.54**	.55**	.59**	.43**	.64**	.65**	.58**	.50**	.45**	.57**

*Significant at the .05 level.
**Significant at the .01 level.

110

Test and the achievement of groups of youngsters should not mislead examiners to assume that such a relationship exists between the schoolwork and the VADS Test performance of each individual pupil. As the present study suggests, the majority of 8- and 10-year-old children who score low (below the 25th percentile) on the VADS Test, especially on the Visual-Oral, Visual Input, and Intersensory Integration measures are also likely to have poor reading recognition, spelling, and arithmetic achievement; this is generally the case, but there are exceptions.

Obviously school achievement depends on many different factors and the VADS Test taps only a small portion of them. Furthermore there are tremendous individual differences between children with learning difficulties. Not all children with low VADS Test scores have problems in reading recognition, nor do all pupils with high VADS Test scores have good reading achievement. Rob, age 9½, is an example of a youngster with high VADS Test and low reading scores. Rob was a pale, thin, sad-looking boy who came from a large, impoverished, socially deprived family. There was a marked discrepancy between his verbal and performance ability (WISC-R Verbal IQ 85, Performance IQ 101, Full Scale IQ 91). He was well coordinated, liked sports, and had good common sense, but his vocabulary was limited and his language skills were weak. He was very concretistic and lacked motivation and intellectual curiosity. Rob received little encouragement or support at home for academic achievement. He did not enjoy reading and did it poorly. He was only able to read second-grade books with effort even though his Total VADS Test score of 26 was superior. His VADS Subtest scores were as follows: Aural-Oral 6, Visual-Oral 7, Aural-Written 6, Visual-Written 7. The high VADS Test performance reflects Rob's good intersensory integration and recall, but it does not reveal his difficulty with sound discrimination and his lack of motivation. Both factors greatly interfered with his reading ability.

Karen presented the opposite picture from Rob. Karen, age 11½, had good reading recognition even though she was only of borderline mental ability (WISC-R Verbal IQ 73, Performance IQ 77, Full Scale IQ 73). Karen was a friendly, attractive, immature, neurologically impaired youngster who was very poorly integrated and was grossly deficient in common sense reasoning ability. She had limited understanding of the world around her and was lacking in social judgment. But Karen had good visual recognition for details and she loved to read. She spent hours each day reading for fun, although she usually did not understand what she read. Her reading recognition was on the fifth-grade level but her reading comprehension was on the first-grade level. Her Total VADS Test score of 18 was on the level of 6½-year-old children. Karen's VADS Subtests were Aural-Oral 4, Visual-Oral 5, Aural-Written 4, Visual-Written 5. Her low VADS Test scores were in keeping with her low academic functioning. They failed to reflect her specific ability for visual recognition. The VADS Test scores measured her poor auditory processing and recall and her poor intersensory integration. Karen read mostly by rote and was unable to integrate and to relate what she read to her daily experiences, and she could not generalize from it. Thus, her reading recognition score was unrealistically high, whereas her VADS Test score concurred with her comprehension level and with her level of social maturity.

SUMMARY

All the VADS Test measures, with the exception of the Aural-Oral Subtest, correlated significantly with the Wide Range Achievement Test scores of 8- and 10-year-old LD pupils. The association of the Reading Recognition, Spelling, and Arithmetic scores was particularly close with the Visual-Oral Subtest and with the Visual Input, Written Expression, Intersensory Integration, and Total VADS Test scores. In addition, The Arithmetic scores were also very closely related to the Visual-Written Subtest.

The correlations between achievement scores and VADS Test measures were higher for LD youngsters than for average public school pupils. Among the LD students there was a closer relationship between Reading, Spelling, and Arithmetic scores and VADS Test scores of the duller 10-year-olds and brighter 8-year-olds than of the brighter 10-year-old and duller 8-year-old LD children.

Chapter 12

VADS Test and IQ Scores

Tables 15 to 22 revealed that the mean VADS Test scores of groups of children with learning difficulties were considerably lower than those of average public school pupils. The extent to which the VADS Test scores differed from the normative scores seemed to depend on the mental ability of the learning-disabled youngsters. At each age level, from 6½ to 14 years, there was a marked discrepancy between the VADS Test mean scores of LD pupils of normal intelligence (WISC IQ 90 or above) and LD pupils of dull normal and borderline mental ability (WISC IQ 70 to 89) and moderately retarded youngsters (WISC IQ 69 or less). Does this mean that the VADS Test is primarily a test of mental ability? In this chapter we examine the relationship of the VADS Test and IQ scores more closely.

In an earlier study (Koppitz, 1970), I investigated the relationship of the VADS Subtests and the IQ scores of two groups of well-functioning elementary school pupils. The IQ scores were derived from the Test of General Ability (TGA) (Flanagan, 1960). Group A consisted of 60 first- to third-graders, and Group B included 40 fourth- and fifth-graders. All of the children were of normal mental ability. Their TGA IQ scores ranged from 89 to 140. The youngsters were divided into four subgroups on the basis of their IQ scores: a) IQ 89 to 109; b) IQ 110 to 119; c) IQ 120 to 129; and d) IQ 130 or more. A comparison of the VADS Subtest scores of the pupils in Group A and Group B with the four different IQ levels was conducted with the help of the Chi-Square statistic. No significant differences were found between various subgroups. Thus, it appears that for well-functioning children of at least average ability the VADS Subtest scores are not able to differentiate between average and above average IQ scores.

In another study (Koppitz, 1973), I also failed to find any significant differences between the VADS Subtest scores of two groups of 9- and 10-year-old boys with emotional and learning problems. One group (N 32) was of average mental ability with a WISC IQ mean of 97 (IQ range of 88 to 109), whereas the other group (N 28) was of low average to borderline mental ability with a WISC IQ mean of 82 (IQ range 71 to 87).

The results of these two studies concur with the findings of Wachs (1969) who studied the ability to recall words in 216 fourth-, eighth-, and twelfth-grade students. One third of the youngsters had low IQ scores of less than 90; another third of the pupils had average IQ scores of 95 to 110; and the remaining third had IQ scores of 115 or more. Wachs reported no significant differences between the recall ability of the average and high IQ groups or between the average and low IQ groups. However, the difference in recall became statistically significant when the extreme groups, that is, the high and low IQ groups were compared.

In the preceding studies, groups of youngsters with a relatively restricted range of IQ scores were compared. The 26 fifth-grade students discussed earlier (see p. 77) represented an entire public school class and showed the usual spread of IQ scores found in a fifth grade of a school located in a lower- to lower-middle-class neighborhood. The Comprehensive Test of Basic Skills (CTBS) had been administered to the youngsters as a group; the test scores revealed a CTBS IQ range from 65 to 130, with an IQ mean score of 95.4. I divided the youngsters into two groups: 14 of them had IQ scores at or above the class mean (IQ 95 to 130), and 12 children had IQ scores below the class mean (IQ 65 to 94).

The pupils with IQ scores above and below the class mean were then compared on all 11 VADS Test measures by means of the Chi-square statistic. As was shown on Table 14, the Visual-Written Subtest and the Visual Input, Oral Expression, Intrasensory Integration, and Total VADS Test scores all showed a significant relationship ($p < .05$) to the CTBS IQ scores. However, the relationship of the VADS Test scores to the Reading, Language, Spelling, and Arithmetic scores was considerably closer than to the IQ scores for this sample of normal fifth-grade pupils.

More recently I correlated the 11 VADS Test scores of learning-disabled pupils with their WISC Verbal, Performance, and Full Scale IQ scores and with their WISC Subtest scores. The 50 subjects for this study were 9-year-old youngsters (CA 9–0 to 9–11) to whom I had previously administered the VADS Test and 11 Subtests of the WISC during routine psychological evaluations. The youngsters included 36 boys and 14 girls, all of whom were enrolled in special public school classes for children with learning disabilities. Their Total VADS Test score mean of 17.5 was at the 10th percentile for 9-year-old children (Appendix A) and below the 10th percentile for third-grade pupils (Appendix B); the score resembled that of 6 years 7-month-old children (Appendix C).

The 50 LD pupils had a WISC Verbal IQ mean of 88 (IQ range 71 to 110), a Performance IQ mean of 97 (IQ range 75 to 125), and a Full Scale IQ mean of 92 (IQ range 75 to 118). The distribution of the WISC Subtest scores was characteristic of many children with learning disabilities (Ackerman et al. 1971; Koppitz, 1971, p. 121). On the Verbal Scale the special class pupils scored highest on the Comprehension and Similarities Subtests, and they had most difficulties with the Digit Span, Arithmetic, and Information Subtests. On the Performance Scale they did best on the Picture Completion and Object Assembly Subtests and scored lowest on the Picture Arrangement and Coding Subtests.

Table 30 represents the reduced correlation matrix between the 11 VADS Test scores and the WISC scores. Since none of the correlations with WISC Comprehension, Similarities, Picture Completion, Picture Arrangement, Block Design, and Object Assembly were significant, they were not included on Table 30. Of the remaining 88 correlations, 19 were not statistically significant, 24 were significant at the .05 level, and 45 were significant at the .01 level.

All 11 VADS Test measures correlated significantly with the WISC

Table 30.

Correlations between VADS Test and WISC Scores[1]

VADS	Verbal IQ	Performance IQ	Full Scale IQ	Information	Arithmetic	Vocabulary	Digit Span	Coding
A–O	.34*	.12	.26	.32*	.13	.21	.61**	.11
V–O	.43**	.23	.36**	.44**	.35**	.32*	.57**	.33*
A–W	.32*	.24	.31*	.31*	.24	.11	.63**	.34*
V–W	.46**	.31*	.42**	.39**	.37**	.36**	.58**	.34*
A I	.36**	.20	.31*	.35**	.20	.18	.69**	.26
V I	.47**	.28*	.41**	.44**	.38**	.36**	.61**	.35**
O E	.43**	.20	.35**	.43**	.28*	.30*	.65**	.26
W E	.43**	.30*	.49**	.38**	.34*	.27*	.65**	.37**
Intra	.46**	.26	.39**	.40**	.30*	.33*	.67**	.27*
Inter	.41**	.25	.36**	.41**	.32*	.25	.65**	.36**
Total	.45**	.26	.39**	.42**	.32*	.30*	.68**	.33*

[1]Correlations between VADS Test and WISC Comprehension, Similarities, Picture Completion, Picture Arrangement, Block Design, and Object Assembly are not given since none of them was statistically significant.

* Significant at the .05 level.

** Significant at the .01 level.

Verbal IQ scores and, with the exception of the Aural-Oral Subtest, with the WISC Full Scale IQ scores. By contrast, only the Visual-Written, Visual Input, and Written Expression Scores correlated significantly with the WISC Performance IQ scores.

As would be expected, the WISC Subtest most closely related to the VADS Test was the Digit Span Test. The WISC Digit Span-Forward is in fact almost identical with the Aural-Oral VADS Subtest, but the WISC Digit Span-Backward has little resemblance to the VADS Test. Witkin (1971) compared the VADS Subtests scores of 272 second-grade pupils with their WISC Digit Span Test performance. The correlations between the Digit Span-Forward and the VADS Subtests were all statistically significant at the .01 level (A-O: $r = .55$; V-O: $r = .30$, A-W: $r = .52$; V-W: $r = .37$). No significant relationship was found between the Digit Span-Backward and the VADS Subtest scores.

Table 30 shows that the WISC Information Subtest also correlated significantly with all 11 VADS Test measures. In addition, the WISC Arithmetic and Vocabulary tests were significantly associated with all VADS Test measures but the Aural-Oral, Aural-Written, and Aural Input scores. Of the six verbal Subtests on the WISC only the Comprehension and Similarities tests failed to show any significant correlations with the VADS Test.

Only one of the five WISC Performance Subtests revealed a statistically significant relationship to the VADS Test, and this was the Coding Subtest. In order to get a good score on the Coding Test a child has to be able to remember the Visual Code so that he will not lose time by having to refer back to the code-key each time he writes a symbol. Thus, the Coding Test is to a large extent a test of visual memory. It comes, therefore, as no surprise that the Coding Test was related to all VADS Test measures that dealt with visual memory and not to the VADS Test measures that involved auditory processing (A-O, A I, OE).

No statistically significant correlations were found between the WISC Picture Completion, Picture Arrangement, Block Design, and Object Assembly Subtests and the VADS Test. None of these tests requires auditory-visual or visual-oral integration or memory since the tests deal exclusively with visual materials that the child has to manipulate.

The results of this study indicated that the VADS Test scores of 9-year-old LD pupils correlated significantly with the three WISC Subtests (Arithmetic, Digit Span, and Coding) that Baumeister and Bartlett (1962) included in the Short Term Memory Factor or Trace Factor. The VADS Test also correlated well with the Information and Vocabulary Tests on the WISC that involve long-term memory. A great many LD children of normal mental ability are quite familiar with the facts and words presented on the Information and Vocabulary Tests but have difficulty recalling their names or meanings. Youngsters with learning problems often told me, in response to test questions: "I know who discovered America," or "I know who invented the light bulb, but I cannot remember his name," or "I know that word but I forgot what it means."

The VADS Test is related to memory and recall but not to common sense and abstract reasoning ability as measured on the WISC Comprehension and Similarities Test. The VADS Test is also not related to visual-motor tasks that do not involve memory, such as the ones included on the WISC Performance Scale, with the exception of the Coding Test. Consequently, the VADS Test does not correlate with the WISC Performance Scale, but is closely related to the WISC Verbal and Full Scale IQ scores.

SUMMARY

The four VADS Subtests are apparently unable to differentiate between groups of youngsters with average and with above average mental ability. But for a group of 9-year-old LD pupils with a wide range of IQ scores (borderling to superior), there was a significant relationship between their WISC and VADS Test scores. The WISC Verbal and Full Scale IQ scores and the WISC Digit Span, Information, Arithmetic, and Vocabulary Subtests correlated significantly with the VADS Test measures. On the Performance Scale only the Coding Subtest was related to the VADS Test. All VADS Test measures, with the exception of Aural-Oral, Aural Input, and Oral Expression correlate significantly with the Coding Test. The WISC Subtests (Information, Arithmetic, Digit Span, and Coding) that contain the largest short-term memory factor are thus most closely related to the VADS Test. The VADS Test can qualify as a brief test of auditory processing and of verbal and written recall, but it does not measure verbal reasoning (WISC Similarities and Comprehension) or the ability to deal with concrete materials and pictures (WISC Picture Completion, Picture Arrangement, Block Design, and Object Assembly).

Chapter 13

Diagnostic Patterns of VADS Test Scores

The VADS Test scores of individual youngsters can be evaluated by comparing these scores with the normative test scores for children of the same age or grade level. Another way of analyzing the VADS Test scores of a given pupil is to look at the test score pattern, that is, to look at the internal consistency of the VADS Test scores and to compare the various scores. The presence of exceptionally high or low VADS Subtest or Combination scores can be diagnostically very significant, although no complete diagnosis can be, or should be, made solely on the basis of the VADS Test score pattern. Furthermore, any evaluation of the VADS Test score pattern has to take a youngster's age, mental ability, and overall functioning level into account.

A low-achieving or slow child may obtain a very poor Total VADS Test score, and yet may reveal one VADS Subtest score that is relatively much higher than the other scores and may reflect a child's specific area of strength. Such exceptional scores can be helpful in suggesting ways in which the youngster can learn and remember best. In the same manner, some pupils of average mental ability who have learning disabilities may show a good overall performance on the VADS Test, although the score of one of the four VADS Subtests may deviate markedly from the other three scores. An unusually low score on one Subtest may reveal a specific weakness that can account in part for the child's learning problems. Such clues can point to the need for a more complete evaluation of a pupil's areas of strengths and difficulties, and can assist in the planning of individualized educational programs and remedial strategies.

We begin by analyzing VADS Test records for exceptionally high or unusually low Subtest scores, and then proceed to explore the diagnostic significance of very high and very low VADS Combination scores.

EXCEPTIONALLY HIGH AURAL-ORAL SCORE

Even very young and immature children who are unable to read and write digits are usually able to repeat some aurally presented digits. Table 7 showed that the Aural-Oral mean scores of 5½- and 6-year-old youngsters was higher than the score mean of the other three VADS Subtests. At age 6½, the Visual-Oral Subtest mean score was slightly higher than the mean of the Aural-Oral Subtest. One can expect, therefore, that the Aural-Oral score will be the highest VADS Subtest score for most kindergarten pupils. Thus, a high Aural-Oral score and lower Visual-Oral, Aural-Written, and Visual-Written Subtest scores usually reflect normal immaturity among school beginners; but when this VADS Test score pattern is found among 7- and 8-

year-olds or among older retarded pupils it could indicate a developmental lag in the child's visual-motor integration, sequencing, and recall.

A somewhat different picture is present when a pupil, age 9 or older, of normal mental ability scores significantly higher on the Aural-Oral Subtest than on the other three VADS Subtests. This occurs relatively rarely and has considerable diagnostic implications. Tommy, age 11 years 2 months represents such a case. Tommy's WISC Full Scale IQ score of 99 (Verbal IQ 94, Performance IQ 104) was average, but Tommy was not an "average" youngster; he was a hypersensitive, quiet boy with severe learning difficulties. He also revealed extremely immature visual-motor perception on the Bender Gestalt Test. After spending four years in a special class for children with learning disabilities, intensive training in visual-motor perception, and remedial reading, Tommy was still functioning in reading and writing only on the end of first-grade level. He knew the letters of the alphabet and their sounds in isolation but had difficulty integrating them. No matter how hard Tommy and his teachers worked, Tommy seemed to be unable to remember which symbol went with which sound and to recall the sequences of symbols and sounds when he was faced with printed words or sentences or when he was asked to write them down.

Tommy's difficulties are clearly reflected on his VADS Test scores: Aural-Oral 6, Visual-Oral 4, Aural-Written 3, and Visual-Written 4. Only the Aural-Oral Subtest score was average for an 11-year-old boy. His memory for visually presented digits (V-O and V-W) and his written recall of digits series (A-W, V-W) were quite defective (below the 10th percentile). Tommy could remember best when he could hear and say the digits. I recommended that Tommy's teachers encourage him to verbalize to himself, either vocally or subvocally, when he read or wrote, so that he could respond to oral stimuli as well as visual ones when he tried to recall a word.

EXCEPTIONALLY LOW AURAL-ORAL SCORE

The Aural-Oral Subtest is the first of the four VADS Subtests presented to a child. Obviously a youngster should always be put at ease before any testing begins. But sometimes a child may still be a bit tense or anxious when the Aural-Oral Subtest is administered. By the time the second VADS Subtest, the Visual-Oral Subtest, is given most pupils are quite relaxed and enjoy the test. Therefore, the Aural-Oral Subtest score may occasionally be somewhat lower than it would have been if the Aural-Oral Subtest had been given later during the test administration. The reason for giving the Aural-Oral Subtest first was outlined in Chapter 3.

It is recommended that the four VADS Subtests be administered in the standardized order, since the VADS Test norms are based on this order. However, I do not believe that a psychologist or diagnostician testing a child should be rigid. When we speak of an exceptionally low Aural-Oral Subtest score, we are assuming that the score is a valid one and that the youngster was doing as well as he was able to do on this particular task. If it is apparent, from the child's subsequent test performance, that he was very tense or did not do as well as he might have done on the Aural-Oral Subtest, then I usually repeat the last digit sequence on the Aural-Oral Subtest that the child previously missed. More often than not the youngster will reproduce the digit sequence again incorrectly, but if he should do significantly better on this second try, then I give him credit for it and let him continue on the subtest until he fails or completes the test. I also make note to the effect that the youngster has a tendency to get anxious and to do poorly when faced with an unfamiliar task or when under pressure; such an observation by itself is of diagnostic value.

For very young and immature children the Aural-Oral Subtest score is almost always the highest one of the four VADS Subtest scores; by age 7 the Visual-Oral Subtest score tends to be slightly higher than the Aural-Oral score. By age 8 both the Visual-Oral and the Visual-Written Subtest scores have usually surpassed the Aural-Oral score; only the Aural-Written Subtest score continues to be lower. Therefore, it is common to find that from age 8 on the Aural-Oral score is lower than at least two of the other VADS Subtest scores. One can only consider an Aural-Oral score exceptionally low when it is at least one point lower than the Aural-Written score and two points lower than the Visual-Oral and Visual-Written Subtest scores.

Sam, age 8 years 2 months, showed this type of VADS Test score pattern. Sam was of average mental ability (WISC Verbal IQ 100, Performance IQ 104, Full Scale IQ 102) and revealed no significant lag in visual-motor perception, to judge from his performance on the Bender Gestalt Test. But Sam's speech and language were quite immature, and he had serious learning disabilities, particularly in the area of reading and spelling. His difficulties with sound-symbol association, sequencing, and recall were reflected on his poor Total VADS Test score of 18. An analysis of Sam's VADS Subtest scores showed that they were in the average range with the exception of the Aural-Oral score, which was below the 10th percentile for 8-year-old children. Sam's VADS Test scores were as follows: Aural-Oral 3, Visual-Oral 5, Aural-Written 5, and Visual-Written 5. It is not surprising that his lowest scores on the WISC were on Arithmetic and Digit Span, which require auditory processing and oral recall. Sam did better on the VADS Subtests when the digit sequences were presented visually and when he could write the digit sequences rather than say them. It appears, therefore, that Sam learned and remembered best that material which he could see and write. His teachers were advised that Sam had great difficulty giving oral reports and remembering what he heard on tapes or in class lectures. For children like Sam, oral instruction should always be accompanied by visual illustrations or manipulative aids.

EXCEPTIONALLY HIGH VISUAL-ORAL SCORE

Of the four VADS Subtests, the Visual-Oral Subtest is most closely related to reading and spelling since it involves the integration of visual symbols with sounds and the recall of visually presented symbol sequences. Most normal youngsters, age 6½ and older, score higher on the Visual-Oral Subtest than on the other three VADS Subtests (Table 7). Therefore, we can only regard a Visual-Oral score as exceptionally high when it is at least two points or more above the scores of the other three Subtests. This was the case with Arlene's Visual-Oral Subtest score.

Arlene obtained a Visual-Oral score of 7, but she had only a score of 5 on the other three VADS Subtests. Her Total VADS Test score of 22 placed her at the 10th percentile of the VADS Test performance for children of her age level. Arlene was 11 years and 2 months old. She was a girl of dull normal mental ability (WISC Verbal IQ 85, Performance IQ 80, and Full Scale IQ 81) with poor abstract reasoning ability. Arlene was a good speller and was able to read (decode) fifth-grade books because of her good visual recognition and recall for symbol sequences, even though she did not understand much of what she read. Her low IQ scores, the poor Total VADS Test score, and her immature Bender Gestalt Test performance were all in keeping with her overall low functioning and with her mental limitations. The high Visual-Oral Subtest score reflected Arlene's specific strength in visual recognition and in visual recall.

EXCEPTIONALLY LOW VISUAL-ORAL SCORE

A very low Visual-Oral Subtest score tends to be of considerable diagnostic significance since the Visual-Oral Subtest score is usually the highest one of the four Subtest scores for school-age children. Most youngsters who score lower on the Visual-Oral Subtest than on the other three Subtests have difficulty with symbol-sound association and with the recognition and recall of visual symbol sequences; they also tend to do poorly in reading and spelling. A very low Visual-Oral Subtest score can often help to pinpoint specific learning disabilities when most other tests and test scores are within the normal range and fail to disclose any serious weaknesses. The case of Vinnie illustrates such a situation.

Vinnie was of normal intelligence (WISC Verbal IQ 104, Performance IQ 113, Full Scale IQ 109) and had good visual-motor perception, as measured on the Bender Gestalt Test. But at age 10 years 10 months, Vinnie was still only reading and spelling on the first grade level. His VADS Test score pattern was most unusual: His Aural-Oral score was 7, the Visual-Oral score was 5, the Aural-Written score was 6, and the Visual-Written score was 6. Thus, Vinnie's Aural-Oral and Aural-Written scores were high average for his age level, and his Visual-Written score was low average; only the Visual-Oral score was defective (10th percentile). His visual and auditory perception were good as was his oral and visual memory. On the WISC, Vinnie obtained a high average score of 12 on both the Digit Span Test (oral memory) and the Coding Test (visual memory). Vinnie suffered from a specific problem in symbol-sound association for letters and in visual memory for symbol sequences. The low Visual-Oral Subtest score reflected these difficulties.

EXCEPTIONALLY HIGH AURAL-WRITTEN SCORE

For most children the Aural-Written Subtest is the most difficult of the four VADS Subtests; it is the VADS Subtest that shows consistently the lowest score mean for youngsters age 5½ to 12 years (Table 7). It is rare to find children who do better on the Aural-Written Subtest than on the other three VADS Subtests. In my extensive collection of VADS Test records of pupils with learning problems I have discovered only a handful of records in which the Aural-Written Subtest was exceptionally high. The youngsters who produced these records had several things in common; they were all of at least average mental ability (WISC IQ 93 to 112), and most of them also showed a marked discrepancy between their Verbal and Performance IQ scores. All of these children were somewhat elusive and withdrawn. Although their auditory perception was perfectly normal, they had difficulty with verbal expression and with visual processing and recall. They were most successful on the Aural-Written Subtest because this test required primarily auditory perception and written expression.

Dave was one of the youngsters who showed this particular VADS Test score pattern. Dave, age 8 years 11 months, had a WISC Verbal IQ of 93, a Performance IQ of 101, and a Full Scale IQ of 99. However, his academic achievement was only on the first-grade level. Dave's Total VADS Test performance was extremely poor, and was in keeping with his school functioning. He obtained a score of 3 on the Aural-Oral, Visual-Oral, and Visual-Written Subtests and a score of 4 on the Aural-Written Subtest. The Aural-Written Subtest score was low average (25th percentile) for 8-year-olds, whereas the other three scores were on the defective level (below the 10th percentile). Dave had serious difficulties with oral expression and with visual memory. He did relatively well with auditory processing and with written recall, and hence with the Aural-Written integration. Dave suffered from an expressive language problem and his visual-motor integration was extremely immature, as could be seen on his Bender Gestalt Test performance. He was a withdrawn and somewhat depressed youngster who rarely participated in class activities.

EXTREMELY LOW AURAL-WRITTEN SCORE

Since it is normal for youngsters to score lower on the Aural-Written Subtest than on the Aural-Oral, Visual-Oral and Visual-Written Subtests (Table 7), a low Aural-Written score has little diagnostic significance unless it is at least two or more points lower than the scores of the other three VADS Subtests. This occurs rather rarely, but one example of this type of VADS Test score pattern was shown on Chrissy's VADS Test record.

Chrissy, age 11 years 6 months, obtained a score of 6 on the Aural-Oral, Visual-Oral, and Visual-Written Subtests, but on the Aural-Written Subtest she had a very low score of only 4 (10th percentile). Chrissy was of average mental ability (WISC Verbal IQ 100, Performance IQ 91, Full Scale IQ 95), but she was extremely impulsive and disorganized; she had difficulty concentrating in class and doing her written assignments. It was particularly difficult for her to process and recall what she heard and to put it down on paper afterward. Chrissy was essentially a visual learner who could give oral reports on what she saw, but had difficulty with writing reports and with spelling. Her school achievement was only on the third-grade level.

EXCEPTIONALLY HIGH VISUAL-WRITTEN SCORE

According to Table 7 the Visual-Written Subtest scores tend to be somewhat lower than the Visual-Oral Subtest scores for young children through age 7. From age 8 on, the magnitude of the Visual-Written scores is usually equal to, or only slightly lower than, the Visual-Oral Subtest scores. It is uncommon to find VADS Test records on which the Visual-Written score is two points higher than the scores of the other three Subtests. However, when this is the case then it has almost always considerable diagnostic implications. If a child's Visual-Written Subtest score is in the average range, and higher than the other VADS Subtest scores, then the other Subtest scores are usually below average, and the child may have difficulty with the processing and recall of what he hears (A-O, A-W), and with the oral expression of what he hears or sees (A-O, V-O); in other words, the youngster may have both receptive and expressive language problems. But a diagnosis of receptive and expressive aphasia can only be made after a complete speech and language evaluation. The VADS Test score pattern can be of help in this process.

Lydia, age 12 years 1 month, was a slow, passive, nonverbal youngster who seemed "turned off" by school and who put forth little effort in the classroom. Her teacher tried to explain Lydia's lack of participation in school activities and her poor achievement by the fact that Lydia came from a Spanish-speaking home. Although she was born in New York City and attended an English-speaking school since kindergarten, Lydia did spend part of each year in Puerto Rico. Both of Lydia's sisters, one older and one younger than Lydia, were good students, outgoing, alert, and fluent in English. The three sisters had essentially the same home background, but only Lydia had difficulty with her schoolwork.

I saw Lydia for a psychological evaluation; she enjoyed the attention she received during the testing session and was very cooperative. Lydia said that she spoke English at home with her sisters and that she counted and dreamed in English. Lydia's performance on the VADS Test was most revealing. Her Total VADS Test score of 18 fell below the 10th percentile for 12-year-olds. She obtained grossly defective scores of 4 on the Aural-Oral, the Visual-Oral, and the Aural-Written Subtests. Lydia's Visual-Written score of 6 was also relatively low for her age level, but it was considerably better than the other three Subtest scores. The VADS Test score pattern suggested that Lydia had very serious difficulties with both auditory processing and with oral expression; that is, Lydia was most likely suffering from a receptive and expressive language disorder. This difficulty appeared to be less a result of her Spanish background than a reflection of probable minimal brain dysfunction.

Lydia's overall functioning was immature and her approach to the VADS Test was primitive. Lydia made no attempt to group or rehearse digits. She was very concretistic and could apparently deal more effectively with material she could see and copy than with language and abstract concepts. This impression was confirmed by her performance on the WISC. Lydia's Verbal IQ score was only 65 or defective, whereas her Performance IQ score was 85. Her Full Scale IQ score was 72. An interview with her parents revealed that Lydia had had a very difficult birth and that her development in early childhood had been slow. Lydia did not begin to walk until she was 2½ years old, and she did not talk until she was 3½ years old. Thus, Lydia was found to be a girl of borderline mental ability with specific problems in receptive and expressive language. Having to cope with two languages and two cultures only added to Lydia's difficulties, but this was not the main cause of her problems. A neurological examination and an EEG both yielded positive findings for Lydia.

EXCEPTIONALLY LOW VISUAL-WRITTEN SCORE

The Visual-Written score of average school beginners tends to be lower than the scores of the other three Subtests. By age 7, the Visual-Written score equals or just surpasses the Aural-Oral Subtest score; thereafter, the Visual-Written score tends to be as high as the Visual-Oral Subtest score (Table 7). Only very young children or retarded youngsters, and some children with learning problems, show exceptionally low Visual-Written Subtest scores. When the Visual-Written score is below average and the scores of the other three VADS Subtests are in the average range, then the youngster reveals the strong likelihood of specific problems or extreme immaturity in visual-motor integration. In such a case, the low Visual-Written score cannot be the result of poor visual perception or poor visual memory since an average score on the Visual-Oral Subtest reflects adequate visual perception and recall. The low Visual-Written score also cannot result from difficulty with writing digits since a fairly good score on the Aural-Written Subtest indicates adequate written recall of digits. A very poor Visual-Written score points, therefore, to specific problems in the integration of visual perception and written expression, or to very poor visual reasoning and learning strategies.

Children who do well on the Visual-Written Subtest tend to verbalize the digit sequences to themselves, either vocally or subvocally, as they read them; in addition, they usually group or chunk the digits to facilitate their recall. As was shown previously, intelligent youngsters spontaneously organize the stimuli and use both auditory and visual clues when writing visual digit sequences from memory. Duller children neither group the digits nor do they verbalize them; they tend to rely entirely on their visual memory. They lack the ability to restructure spontaneously and simplify the task for themselves; they have to be specifically taught how to do this. Many dull children and pupils with learning problems tend to be rigid and need to be "pointed" or cued in to alternative or simpler ways of solving problems.

Diane, age 10 years 11 months, was one of these dull youngsters (WISC Verbal IQ score 82, Performance IQ score 68, Full Scale IQ score 73) with serious difficulties in visual-motor integration and recall. Her VADS Test scores were Aural-Oral 6, Visual-Oral 5, Aural-Written 5, and Visual-Written 3. Thus, her processing of aurally presented digits (A-O, A-W) was average (50th percentile) for 10-year-olds; the Visual-Oral score was low (10th percentile), whereas the Visual-Written score was grossly defective (below the 10th percentile). It seems that Diane was better able to sequence and recall visual stimuli when she could repeat them orally; when the task did not specifically require this Diane could not evoke auditory associations from visual stimuli. She remained rigidly bound to the input information. Her immature visual-motor integration was also reflected in her very poor Bender Gestalt Test performance. Academically Diane was functioning only at the beginning first-grade level.

DIAGNOSTIC PATTERNS OF VADS COMBINATION SCORES

So far we have only evaluated the diagnostic significance of exceptionally high or exceptionally low VADS Subtest scores. It was shown previously that the VADS Combination scores have a higher correlation with school achievement than do the four Subtest scores. It stands to reason that the VADS Combination score patterns would also have greater diagnostic value for the assessment of learning problems than the score patterns of the four Subtests. We therefore explore at this time the relationship of learning difficulties to very high and very low Aural Input and Visual Input scores, to exceptionally good and exceptionally poor Oral Expression and Written Expression, and to outstanding and defective Intrasensory Integration and Intersensory Intergration.

The assessment of the Combination scores has to take the youngsters age, mental ability, and general functioning into consideration. Obviously no diagnosis can be solely based on VADS Test scores, but the VADS Combination scores can offer suggestions and point the way to areas of competence and to possible problems that need to be either confirmed or ruled out. Discrepancies between the Combination scores can reveal children's preferred style of learning. The VADS Combination score patterns can be, therefore, exceedingly helpful in the planning of individualized learning programs and remedial lessons for pupils with specific learning disabilities.

HIGH AURAL INPUT SCORE, LOW VISUAL INPUT SCORE

Table 7 shows that, from age 6½ on, the Visual Input scores (V-O & V-W) are consistently higher than the Aural Input scores (A-O & A-W). A markedly higher (two points or more) Aural Input score than Visual Input score on the VADS Test therefore suggests a weakness or problem in visual processing and recall. Since the Aural Input and Visual Input scores both include oral and written expression, the difference between the two scores has to result from the mode of input rather than from the mode of output. Large discrepancies between the Aural Input and Visual Input scores can occur at all age levels and among bright as well as among dull children. Thus, such a discrepancy could involve an outstanding Aural Input score as compared with a Visual Input score that was only average, or it could involve an average or even low Aural Input score while the Visual Input score was extremely low or defective.

The children who score significantly higher on VADS Aural Input than on Visual Input are most likely auditory learners and may need special help with visual processing, integration, and recall. I analyzed the VADS Test records of 17 LD pupils who showed a much higher (two points or more) Aural Input score than Visual Input score. The youngsters, who ranged in age from 7½ to 12, included eight boys and nine girls. Most of them were of borderline or dull normal mental ability (IQ score mean 80) and functioned on the first-grade level. They had very immature visual-motor perception, as measured on the Bender Gestalt Test (Bender Test mean 7.8). One of this group was Stephanie.

Stephanie was an immature, deprived, 9½-year-old girl of borderline mental ability (WISC Verbal IQ score 75, Performance IQ score 83, Full Scale IQ score 77). She was quite verbal and showed good social skills; however, she was very concretistic and had extremely poor perceptual-motor integration. This was reflected on the VADS Test and on the Bender Gestalt Test. On both tests Stephanie functioned barely on the 5-year-old level. Of particular interest were her VADS Test scores: Aural-Oral 4, Visual-Oral 3, Aural-Written 4, and Visual-Written 3. The test scores show that Stephanie's Total VADS score of 14 and her overall perceptual-motor integration, sequencing, and recall were very low (below 10th percentile), but her processing of aurally presented digits was relatively much better than was her processing of visually presented stimuli. Stephanie was better able to learn and to remember what she heard than what she saw; she needed verbal instructions as well as specific training in visual-motor perception. Stephanie needed help with visual analysis, tracing of shapes, visual tracking, and in forming auditory associations with visual stimuli. Since she could recall oral information better than visual stimuli, Stephanie needed to be encouraged to verbalize to herself, either vocally or subvocally, what she tried to read and write.

HIGH VISUAL INPUT SCORE, LOW AURAL INPUT SCORE

From age 6 on, (Table 7) average schoolchildren tend to score higher on VADS Visual Input (V-O & V-W) than on Aural Input (A-O & A-W). Therefore, a Visual Input score that is only slightly higher (one or two points) than the Aural Input score must be considered normal; it has no diagnostic significance. Only when the Visual Input score is at least three or more points greater than the Aural Input score can we say that the Visual Input score is significantly higher than the Aural Input score, and only then does it have diagnostic implications.

Of the LD sample 51 VADS Test records revealed a significant discrepancy between the Visual Input and Aural Input scores. In each case the discrepancy resulted from an unusually low Aural Input score rather than from an exceptionally high Visual Input score. That is, the youngsters showed a marked weakness in auditory processing and in the sequencing and recall of heard digit sequences. Most of the children were of average or low average mental ability, and most had higher WISC Performance IQ scores than Verbal IQ scores. WISC IQ score means for this group were Verbal 84.4, Performance 95.2, and Full Scale 88.6.

The 51 pupils fell into two different groups. The majority not only had learning difficulties but were also restless, explosive, and in many cases acting-out youngsters, whereas the others were quiet and withdrawn. The description of two LD pupils illustrates the two types of youngsters with high Visual Input scores and low Aural Input scores. One of the pupils was Barry, an acting-out youngster, whereas the other, Mel, was quite withdrawn.

Barry, a bright 8½-year-old, was extremely restless, hyperactive, distractible; his frustration tolerance was very low, and he talked incessantly. Yet, his speech was slurry and his language was quite immature. He mispronounced words and used incorrect sentence structures. Despite good intelligence and mental curiosity, Barry was unable to concentrate; he rarely participated in class discussion or completed his assignments. His teacher complained that Barry "never listened," or remembered what he was told. When Barry was not engrossed in drawing violent pictures, he disrupted and annoyed other children. Barry had little love for school; he had experienced continuous failure and frustration in his classes, starting with kindergarten.

I observed Barry in class; his behavior convinced me that he really could not sit still and follow class discussions, though he could read and comprehend third-grade books with ease. However, Barry did not share with others what he had read. He had become discouraged and angry with his teacher and school; he lacked self-confidence. More often than not he did not even try to do his work and could not tolerate when other children did their work. His acting-out behavior reflected his frustration and anger.

When I gave Barry a psychological evaluation he enjoyed the attention he received and was challenged by the tests as long as they were not related to school achievement. He was threatened by anything that reminded him of schoolwork and failure. He liked the VADS Test and put forth much effort while taking it. The VADS Test scores were quite revealing: Aural-Oral score 4, Visual-Oral 6, Aural-Written 4, and Visual-Written 6. Thus, his Aural Input score (A-O & A-W) was 8 as compared to a score of 12 on Visual Input (V-O & V-W). The Visual Input score was high average for 8-year-olds (Appendix A), whereas the Aural Input score was quite poor and only at the

10th percentile. The VADS Test results are consistent with Barry's WISC scores: his Verbal IQ was 105, his Performance IQ was 120. Barry also displayed very poor auditory sequencing and recall on the WISC (Digit Span score 6), but his memory for visual symbols was good (Coding score 12).

There could be no doubt that Barry was a bright youngster with good verbal and visual reasoning (WISC Similarities score 13, Block Design score 16), but he was a vulnerable, poorly controlled boy who had specific difficulties in auditory processing and recall. He really did find it hard to follow group discussions and to remember verbal instructions. This, of course, greatly interfered with his schoolwork. His parents and his teacher were aware of Barry's good mental ability, but they failed to recognize his very real areas of weakness. They expected more from Barry than he was able to achieve. Constant failure resulted in much frustration, anger, and a negative attitude toward school. This, in turn, only reinforced Barry's poor achievement. Barry obviously had emotional and behavior problems when I saw him, but the VADS Test results clearly reflect his underlying problems in auditory processing.

Mel was a battered child who had been removed from his home when he was 3 years old, and had been placed into a foster home. When I tested Mel he was 14 years 10 months old. He obtained exactly the same scores on the VADS Test as Barry did. Mel also had an Aural Input score of 8 and a Visual Input score of 12. But since Mel was 14½ years old a Visual Input score of 12 was quite low, and an Aural Input score of 8 was grossly defective. Mel was an emotionally and socially deprived youngster with severe problems in auditory perception and language skills. He had difficulty understanding verbal instructions and he had serious speech problems. Mel was quiet and withdrawn; he rarely spoke and had difficulty relating to his peers. Most of the time he sat by himself and drew pictures. His academic skills were quite poor and he functioned barely on the third-grade level in reading and arithmetic.

Mel's VADS Test record corresponded to his WISC IQ scores. His Verbal IQ score was only 88, whereas his Performance IQ score was 100. Mel was a youngster with multiple problems, including a severe handicap in auditory perception that was reflected on his VADS Test performance. His severe language problem could probably be traced back to his traumatic early history. When I saw Mel for testing he was at ease and very responsive. In fact, Mel enjoyed the testing session and wanted to come again. The poor VADS Test performance was not the result of undue anxiety or lack of effort on his part; rather it reflected a serious problem with auditory processing.

HIGH ORAL EXPRESSION SCORE, LOW WRITTEN EXPRESSION SCORE

At all age levels, from 5½ to 12 years, the VADS Oral Expression scores (A-O & V-O) tend to be higher than the Written Expression scores (A-W & V-W). For very young children this difference is considerable. The Oral

Expression score mean for the 5½-year-old normative sample was 7.7, whereas the Written Expression score mean was only 5.8 (Table 7). The magnitude of the discrepancy between the two tests decreases as the pupils get older, but even with normal 12-year-olds the Oral Expression score tends to be somewhat higher than the Written Expression score. Therefore, a difference of one or even two points between the Oral Expression and the Written Expression scores on an individual child's VADS Test record cannot usually be regarded as diagnostically significant; a difference of three or more points on the other hand has considerable diagnostic implications, especially among brighter and older youngsters.

A significant discrepancy between the Oral and Written Expression scores results most often from a difficulty with written expression. School-age children who know numbers and who do well on VADS Oral Expression but poorly on Written Expression usually reveal specific problems with fine-motor coordination. I found that a group of 13 LD pupils with a significantly higher (three points or more) Oral Expression than Written Expression score also had higher WISC Verbal IQ scores than Performance IQ scores. The results showed that the children had not only poor writing but they also had difficulty manipulating puzzles and blocks. Anthony, age 7 years and 7 months, and Ted, age 12 years 11 months, belonged to this group of youngsters.

Anthony's teacher was concerned about him and asked for a psychological evaluation. Anthony appeared to be bright, but he rebelled against doing any written work and, when the teacher was not watching him, he would disappear from the classroom. The teacher found him repeatedly hiding in the coat closet, under the staircase, or out on the playground. Anthony told me that he hated school. He complained, "I get tired, too much work, too much writing." Anthony was a sensitive, tall, awkward youngster who tripped over his own feet when he walked and had difficulty holding and controlling a pencil. But he was alert and loved to read.

Anthony was very responsive during the testing session; he worked slowly and deliberately, putting forth a great deal of effort. I administered the VADS Test first. Anthony's approach to the test showed good intelligence; his test scores were quite revealing. He obtained a score of 6 on the Aural-Oral Subtest, a score of 7 on the Visual-Oral test, and a score of 5 on both the Aural-Written and Visual-Written Subtests. He did extremely well on the first two Subtests and earned an exceptionally high (90th percentile) score of 13 in Oral Expression. By contrast, his performance on the Aural-Written and Visual-Written Subtests was exceedingly laborious and his Written Expression score of 10 was only average (50th percentile) for his age level. It was apparent that the process of writing required so much energy on his part that Anthony forgot some of the digits before he could write them down. Writing was a very difficult task for him; he needed much more time for this effort than most children. Despite his efforts his numbers were misshapen, uneven in size, and poorly spaced.

After the VADS Test I administered the Bender Gestalt Test to Anthony. This proved to be an even harder task for him than the VADS Test had been and Anthony showed visible signs of fatigue. He required twice as long as most youngsters his age to complete the Bender Test, and the results were extremely poor. He got very frustrated when he could not draw the angles, curves, and proportions of a design. His Bender Test score of 11 resembled that of a 5-year-old child. When a child has difficulty with both the VADS Written Expression and the Bender Gestalt Test while his Oral Expression score is good, then he is bound to have poor motor coordination but good visual perception.

Anthony showed a significant discrepancy on the WISC between his Verbal IQ of 113 and his Performance IQ of 97, and between oral reading (grade level score 3.9) and writing and spelling (grade level score 2.4). The test results indicated that Anthony was correct; the teacher had demanded too much work and too much writing from him. He really did get exhausted when he had to write or draw for more than a few minutes. I had to divide the testing sessions into several short periods in order to get maximum performance from Anthony. Anthony was so poorly coordinated that he had to exert enormous energy whenever he used his hands. Since he was bright, he was painfully aware of his difficulties and his inability to perform up to his own standards. He tried to avoid written work altogether and withdrew from his class rather than experience repeated failure and disapproval.

Based on the test results and observations, an individualized program was worked out for Anthony. He was allowed to dictate his book reports and was given each day a short period of intensive visual-motor training and practice in writing. All written assignments were made very brief and he was given as much time as he needed to complete the tasks.

Ted, age 12½ years, was the other youngster with high Oral Expression and low Written Expression scores. He was of essentially average mental ability (WISC Verbal IQ score 96, Performance IQ score 83, Full Scale IQ score 89). Ted was especially interested in social studies and participated actively in class discussions. Ted was a verbal youngster, but he rarely completed his written assignments. When he did write a report it was almost illegible and extremely poor. Ted could read sixth-grade books with comprehension but his writing and spelling were barely on the third- to fourth-grade level. Though tall and fairly good at sports Ted had poor fine-muscle coordination and writing was hard for him.

Ted worked very slowly on the Bender Gestalt Test. With considerable effort on his part he was able to copy the nine Bender Test designs with only one minor imperfection. His Bender Test score of 1 reflects in no way Ted's very real problem with written expression. As was pointed out previously, most normal 10-year-old children are able to reproduce the Bender Test figures correctly so that a score of 1 merely indicated that, at age 12½, Ted was able to copy designs as well as most fifth-graders. The way Ted went about drawing the figures was more revealing than the Bender Test score. For pupils of Ted's age the VADS Test scores tend to be diagnostically more meaningful than the Bender Test scores.

On the VADS Test, Ted obtained the following scores: Aural-Oral 6, Visual-Oral 7, Aural-Written 5, and Visual-Written 4. His Total VADS Test score of 22 was low (10th percentile), indicating that Ted's general perceptual-motor integration, sequencing, and recall was poor. But the analysis of his VADS Test score pattern shows a considerable unevenness and specific areas of strength and weakness. There was a marked discrepancy between Ted's average Oral Expression score of 13 and his defective score of 9 in Written Expression. The VADS Test showed quite clearly that he had serious problems with writing. Every effort was made to make his teachers aware of his problems, and to urge them·to reduce the amount of written work they would expect from Ted, and to allow more time for him to complete his assignments. In a meeting with Ted and his teachers it was jointly decided that it would be better for Ted to complete a somewhat shorter assignment than to be overwhelmed by a long assignment with which he could not cope. His social studies teacher permitted Ted to write only brief reports and to supplement these with projects and oral reports.

HIGH WRITTEN EXPRESSION SCORE, LOW ORAL EXPRESSION SCORE

It is relatively rare to find children whose Written Expression score (A-W & V-W) is significantly higher (two or more points) than their Oral Expression score (A-O & V-O). As was indicated previously, most pupils, age 5½ to 12 years, score higher on Oral Expression than on Written Expression; therefore, it is diagnostically important when a VADS Test record displays a higher score on Written Expression than on Oral Expression. This type of VADS Test score pattern tends to reveal a specific weakness or problem in expressive language, especially if both VADS Subtests included in Written Expression (A-W & V-W) are higher than both Subtests included in Oral Expression (A-O & V-O).

Scott was one of the 13 LD youngsters who showed this type of VADS Test score pattern. Scott was a shy, insecure, nonverbal boy of average mental ability (WISC Verbal IQ score 96, Performance IQ score 94, and Full Scale IQ score 95). I met Scott the first time when he was 7 years old. He was then very small, immature, timid, and never talked in school. When he was 9 years 11 months, I gave him a psychological evaluation at the request of his classroom teacher. The teacher wanted to know whether Scott was retarded. He still rarely spoke in class and his achievement was negligible.

Scott proved to be very cooperative during the testing session, even though he was unspontaneous. Of particular interest was his VADS Test performance. Scott's VADS Test scores were Aural-Oral 4, Visual-Aural 4, Aural-Written 5, and Visual-Written 5. His Total VADS Test score of 18 was quite low for a 9-year-old boy and resembled the score of 6½-year-old children (Appendix B). Thus, Scott's overall perceptual-motor integration and recall were poor and could explain in part his limited reading and writing ability. An analysis of Scott's VADS Test score pattern showed an average score on Written Expression and a defective score (below 10th percentile) on Oral Expression. The VADS Test performance indicated therefore that Scott was a youngster with general problems in sequencing and memory, and with specific problems in oral expression.

When I talked to Scott and listened to his verbal responses to test questions, it became apparent that he had indeed a severe expressive language disorder. He groped for words, spoke in a whisper, and used incorrect grammar. Yet, his auditory perception was good. Scott had no difficulty following verbal instructions and he did not mispronounce words. Scott's reasoning was also adequate, but he had trouble putting his thoughts into words; it was easier for him to write his thoughts or to illustrate them with drawings. Poor memory together with difficulty in oral expression proved to be a great handicap and seriously interfered with Scott's progress in school. He appeared to be much duller than he really was since he could not remember much of what he learned, and even when he knew answers he had difficulty verbalizing them. Scott was not a retarded youngster, but a boy of average mental ability with severe language disabilities and learning problems for which he needed help.

HIGH INTRASENSORY INTEGRATION, LOW INTERSENSORY INTEGRATION

As shown on Table 7, groups of public school children, age 5½ to 12, tend to score somewhat higher on Intrasensory Integration (A-O & V-W) than on Intersensory Integration (V-O & A-W). This is especially true for very young and immature pupils. Rudel and Teuber (1971) obtained similar results in their studies with intramodal and intermodal transfer tasks. Very young children find it easier to work within one sense modality than to have to switch from one sense modality to another or to integrate different sense modalities. For instance, they may be able to repeat what they hear and copy designs or symbols they can look at, but they may have difficulty when they have to follow verbal directions when drawing or when they have to report orally on what they see.

For most school-age youngsters the VADS Intrasensory Integration and Intersensory Integration scores differ only by one scoring point; often the scores are even the same. Only when the Intrasensory Integration score is two or more points higher than the Intersensory Integration score is the difference of diagnostic importance. Such a discrepancy could reflect either a developmental lag or a specific disability in Intersensory Integration. A high Intrasensory Integration score is usually accompanied by an unusually low Intersensory Integration score.

Of the 23 LD pupils with a high Intrasensory Integration score and an unusually low Intersensory Integration score the majority had also differences of 10 or more points between their Verbal and Performance IQ scores on the WISC. Some of the children had higher Verbal IQ scores, others had higher Performance IQ scores. The common characteristic of all 23 youngsters with poor VADS Intersensory Integration scores was uneven functioning and many inconsistencies in their behavior. A well-functioning pupil can integrate new material with what he has learned before, and can relate one type of experience or perception to another type of perception or experience. A child with problems in Intersensory Integration has difficulty doing this.

Doug, age 9 years 5 months, and Jim, age 11 years 6 months, were two LD youngsters who displayed markedly higher Intrasensory Integration scores than Intersensory Integration scores on the VADS Test. They both had areas of outstanding strengths and weaknesses, but they both functioned so unevenly that they required highly individualized educational programs. Both youngsters had been unable to get along in regular classes and were attending special classes for children with learning disabilities. Both were very poor students and were highly atypical. Aside from these similarities, Doug and Jim differed greatly from each other.

After failing both the first and the second grade, Doug had become extremely frustrated and had displayed behavior problems as well as serious learning difficulties. When he was transferred to a special class for learning-disabled pupils, Doug relaxed and developed into a hard-working, enthusiastic pupil who had perfect school attendance. Doug loved school as long as he could work with instructional material that was geared to the interest level of an 8- to 9-year-old boy but that required only first-grade reading skills. Despite average mental ability (WISC Verbal IQ score 91, Performance IQ score 106, Full Scale IQ score 98) Doug was practically a nonreader. He knew all the letters and sounds in isolation but seemed unable to integrate the two; when faced with a word or sentence Doug could not remember which symbol belonged to which sound; moreover, he mixed up their sequences in words. Doug had a severe problem with integrating information that involved more than one sense modality.

Doug's problems were clearly demonstrated on his VADS Test performance. His VADS Test scores were Aural-Oral 5, Visual-Oral 4, Aural-Written 4, and Visual-Written 5. His Total VADS Test score of 18 was quite low (15th percentile) for 9-year-old children. His Intrasensory Integration score of 10 was low average (25th percentile), whereas his Intersensory Integration score of 8 was quite defective and fell below the 10th percentile for children of his age level (Appendix A). Doug's overall ability for sequencing and recall was somewhat immature, but in addition he had specific problems in the integration of visual and auditory stimuli. He worked best when the stimuli and the mode of expression were in the same sense modality; that is, either all auditory (A-O) or all visual (V-W).

Particularly noteworthy was Doug's positive attitude toward school and school learning despite his serious learning problems. Much of the credit for this had to go to Doug's accepting parents, to his teachers, and to Doug's own personality structure. I have observed that many poorly integrated children live in the present and do not dwell on the past or on the future; they live each day as a distinct event and often fail to relate or integrate the experience of the moment with past or future experiences. It is not uncommon to find that poorly integrated children act differently in different situations; they react mainly to the moment. In the regular class Doug had been overwhelmed and frustrated and had developed serious behavior problems. He adjusted well to the small, highly structured class for children with learning disabilities; Doug was happy and secure in the special class. As a consequence, he worked hard and behaved exceptionally well in this supportive setting.

The other poorly integrated youngster with serious learning problems was Jim. In many ways Jim was the exact opposite of Doug. Where Doug had a severe memory deficit for symbols and sounds and was unable to read, Jim had a superb memory for facts and figures and was an excellent reader. He devoured the encyclopedia and the World Almanac and had a prodigious fund of esoteric information. Jim just could not understand why his classmates did not share his enthusiasm when he told them in detail about the per capita income of the inhabitants of Katmandu, the exact amount of annual rainfall in Rumania, or the average life span of the Fiji Islanders. When Jim was questioned about his knowledge, it was evident that he had little comprehension of what the figures he had memorized meant.

Jim had very little understanding of the world around him; where Doug had excelled in common sense reasoning and social judgment, Jim grossly lacked both common sense and social judgment. Jim was unable to integrate his various perceptions and his vast amount of factual information into meaningful relationships and experiences. Abstract reasoning was difficult for him. In fact, Jim was a rather dull youngster. His WISC Verbal IQ score of 91 was spuriously high because of his good memory and large vocabulary. His Performance IQ score was only 74, and his Full Scale IQ score was 81. As with many poorly integrated youngsters, there was a considerable discrepancy between Jim's Verbal and Performance IQ scores. Jim also had difficulty relating to his peers; he was a social isolate.

In view of Jim's excellent memory, I had anticipated that he would do extremely well on the VADS Test; but this was not the case. His VADS Test scores were Aural-Oral 6, Visual-Oral 5, Aural-Written 5, and Visual-Written 7. Jim's Total VADS Test score of 23 was only low average (25th percentile) for 11-year-old children (Appendix A). The VADS Test score pattern was diagnostically very revealing and reflected both Jim's strength and weakness. His Intrasensory Integration score of 13 was high average (75th percentile), whereas his Intersensory Integration score of 10 was very poor (10th percentile). Thus, it appeared that Jim had good memory for what he heard and for what he saw, but had great difficulty integrating the visual with the oral and the auditory with the visual, just as he had problems with the integration of all the bits of information he memorized, and with making sense out of his various experiences. For Jim, life consisted of a multitude of disconnected facts, figures, and sensations.

HIGH INTERSENSORY INTEGRATION, LOW INTRASENSORY INTEGRATION

It is unusual for average schoolchildren, age 5½ to 12, to score markedly higher (two or more points) on Intersensory Integration (V-O & A-W) than on Intrasensory Integration (A-O & V-W). Table 7 shows that the Intrasensory Integration scores of groups of pupils tend to be somewhat higher than the

Intersensory Integration scores. Among the LD sample were 12 youngsters who did not conform to the usual VADS Test score pattern. Their Intersensory Integration scores were significantly higher than their Intrasensory Integration scores. These children differed greatly from the LD pupils discussed previously with high Intrasensory Integration and low Intersensory Integration scores.

As a group the 12 LD youngsters were rather dull (WISC Full Scale IQ score mean 82.8) and their achievement was very low. The most outstanding characteristic of these children was their rigidity, lack of flexibility, and poor adaptability.

The VADS Test records of these LD pupils were most revealing. Their overall functioning in perceptual-motor integration, sequencing, and recall was quite poor, and their Total VADS Test scores were extremely low. Most of the Total VADS scores fell below the 10th percentile. The Intrasensory Integration scores were even lower than the Total VADS Test scores. The very poor Intrasensory Integration score indicated that the youngsters had particular difficulty with the Aural-Oral and Visual-Written Subtests.

A good performance on the Aural-Oral Subtest requires that the children restructure and simplify the task by grouping or chunking the digits. A good performance on the Visual-Written Subtest presupposes that the pupils verbalize the digits, either vocally or subvocally, and group them to facilitate their recall as the youngsters write them down. Both of these strategies are usually used by children who are flexible and have good reasoning ability. School-age children who do not spontaneously group and rehearse the digit sequences tend to get low scores on the Aural-Oral and Visual-Written Subtests. Rigid youngsters are rarely able to restructure the tasks on the Aural-Oral and Visual-Written Subtests on their own. In consequence, they also most often get low scores on these Subtests.

Many rigid pupils do better on the Intersensory Integration Subtest (V-O & A-W) than on the Intrasensory Integration Subtest because the Visual-Oral and Aural-Written Subtests involve the integration of stimuli and responses in two different sense modalities. The tasks of these two Subtests dictate the use of both the visual and the auditory sense modalities. It is not that the rigid youngsters are unable to integrate the visual with the oral, or the oral with the visual; rather they have difficulty knowing when to do so, and how to generalize from one task or experience to another. Very young, or dull and rigid children lack the ability to devise learning strategies on their own; when the pupils are taught how to use learning strategies in a specific situation they are usually successful in following the directions. However, they tend to have difficulty remembering and applying the learning strategies to different situations at a later date.

One such rigid LD pupil was Timmy, age 10 years 1 month. Timmy was a cheerful, good-natured, well-motivated youngster who was eager to please. After an assignment had been explained to Timmy in great detail, he worked willingly and patiently until it was completed. But if Timmy was presented with a task that was new, or when he did not receive explicit instructions, then Timmy was at a loss where to begin. He could not generalize from what he had learned. Timmy was exceedingly rigid and his reasoning was quite poor. On the WISC Timmy obtained a Verbal IQ score of only 79, a Performance IQ score of 87, and a Full Scale IQ score of 81. Despite hard work and a great desire to succeed, Timmy was functioning academically only at the end-of-second-grade level.

Timmy's VADS Test scores were Aural-Oral 5, Visual-Oral 6, Aural-Written 6, and Visual-Written 5. His Total VADS Test score of 22 was low average (25th percentile) for his age level (Appendix A). Timmy's Intersensory Integration score of 12 was average (50th percentile) for 10-year-olds, whereas his score of 10 on Intrasensory Integration was very low (10th percentile). Timmy made no attempt to group the digits either on the Aural-Oral Subtest or on the Visual-Written Subtest. He also did not verbalize or rehearse the visually presented digit sequences since he was not specifically directed to do so. On the Visual-Oral Subtest Timmy had to verbalize the visually presented digits. Therefore he did better on that Subtest than on the Visual-Written Subtest. His performance on the VADS Test corresponded to his behavior in the classroom. Timmy was the kind of youngster who did well on a routine job when he could diligently follow a set assignment without having to make any changes or having to make any decisions about the course of action to take.

DIAGNOSTIC PATTERNS OF VADS TEST SCORES: SUMMARY

In addition to comparing children's VADS Test scores with the normative data, the VADS Test score patterns of individual pupils can also be analyzed. An unusually high or low VADS Subtest score that differs markedly from the other three Subtest scores is usually diagnostically very revealing. The same is true for a significant discrepancy between the Aural Input score and the Visual Input score, between the Oral Expression score and the Written Expression score, and between Intrasensory Integration and Intersensory Integration scores. The diagnostic implications for each such VADS Test score pattern were discussed in detail and illustrated by means of VADS Test records and histories of LD pupils.

Chapter 14

Application of the VADS Test

The VADS Test was primarily designed to serve two purposes: as a clinical tool to help diagnose specific learning problems in schoolchildren, and as a quick and easy-to-use instrument for the screening of school beginners for potential learning difficulties. This chapter illustrates how the VADS Test can be applied as a diagnostic tool for individual pupils and as part of a screening battery for end-of-kindergarten children.

Different ways of analyzing the VADS Test performances of schoolchildren were discussed in detail in the preceding chapters. It was pointed out that the examiner can observe the children's attitudes and behavior while the youngsters are taking the VADS Test, and that the VADS Test records can be evaluated for the quality of the written digits and for the organization of the digit sequences on paper. Normative data were presented so that pupils' VADS Test scores could be compared with the scores of a representative sample of other children of the same age (Appendix A) or grade level (Appendix C); youngsters' functional level could be determined by comparing their VADS Test scores with equal scores of the normative sample (Appendix B). The diagnostic implications of different VADS Test score patterns were spelled out. Each of these different aspects of the VADS Test was examined separately.

The manner in which all of these different approaches to the VADS Test can be integrated and applied to the VADS Test performance of individual children can now be demonstrated. Ten case histories are presented to show the large amount of information that can be obtained when using the VADS Test as a clinical instrument. The youngsters whose case histories are discussed were all children whom I had seen for psychological evaluation because of their learning and behavior problems, or who were enrolled in special public school classes for pupils with learning disabilities.

1. CASE HISTORY: JASON

Jason, age 7 years 8 months, had just lost his first front tooth; he looked like an immature six-year-old child. He was small for his age, hypersensitive, and anxious, but he appeared to be alert and was quite talkative. Despite good mental ability (WISC-R Verbal IQ score 117, Performance IQ score 95, Full Scale IQ score 107), Jason was unable to function in a large, regular class. He was very distractible, disorganized, and worked from right to left. His academic skills were limited; he could only recognize a few letters, write his name, and add and subtract numbers from 1 to 5 by counting on his fingers.

Jason was very cooperative during the administration of the VADS Test and he put forth effort. The test results are considered to be a valid measure of his level of functioning.

On the *Aural-Oral Subtest* Jason was able to repeat the three- and four-digit series correctly but missed both trials on the five-digit series. He had difficulty with the sequencing of the digits, and he substituted some incorrect digits. *His A-O score was 4.*

On the *Visual-Oral Subtest* Jason recalled correctly the three- and four-digit series; he missed the first five-digit sequence, but he repeated the second five-digit sequence without error. Jason missed both six-digit sequences as a result of errors in sequencing and substitutions. *Thus, his V-O score was 5.*

Before administering the *Aural-Written Subtest,* I asked Jason to write the digits from 1 to 9 across the top of the page. As can be seen on Plate 27, Jason reversed the 6, 7, and 9. This is quite unusual for a 7½-year-old child of average mental ability (Table 2), and suggests specific problems with directionality.

When I presented the first three-digit series (532), Jason wrote 531, but quickly corrected himself by writing a 2 over the 1. The first four-digit series was 5826. Jason wrote 586, inverting the 6. When he became aware that he had omitted a digit, he tried to correct his error by writing a 2 over the 6 instead of in front of it; he then added a 1 at the end of the sequence. Jason was able to write the second four-digit sequence correctly but again reversed the 9 and the 7. The process of sequencing, recalling, and writing the digits required a great deal of concentration and energy from Jason. He visibly tired and was no longer able to concentrate on the five-digit series. Thus, he wrote 17628 almost at random, substituting digits, placing others in the wrong sequences, and reversing two of them. After that Jason gave up. *His A-W score was 4.*

On the *Visual-Written Subtest* Jason was able to recall correctly the three-digit series of 538. Thereafter he was unable to reproduce any more digit sequences. He did not remember the sequences long enough to write them down. Jason was fatigued and needed a period of rest and a change of activity. He might have been able to write a four-digit series if he had been given another chance later on, but his short attention span and the fact that he tired so quickly was diagnostically significant and gave a good picture of his functioning in school. Because of this, Jason's Visual-Written score was recorded on the basis of his actual test performance. *His V-W score was 3.*

Thus Jason's VADS Test scores were:

VADS	Score	Percentile	VADS	Score	Percentile
A–O	4	10 to 25	A I	8	10 to 25
V–O	5	25 to 50	V I	8	10
A–W	4	10 to 25	O E	9	25
V–W	3	below 10	W E	7	below 10
Total	16	10	Intra	7	below 10
			Inter	9	25

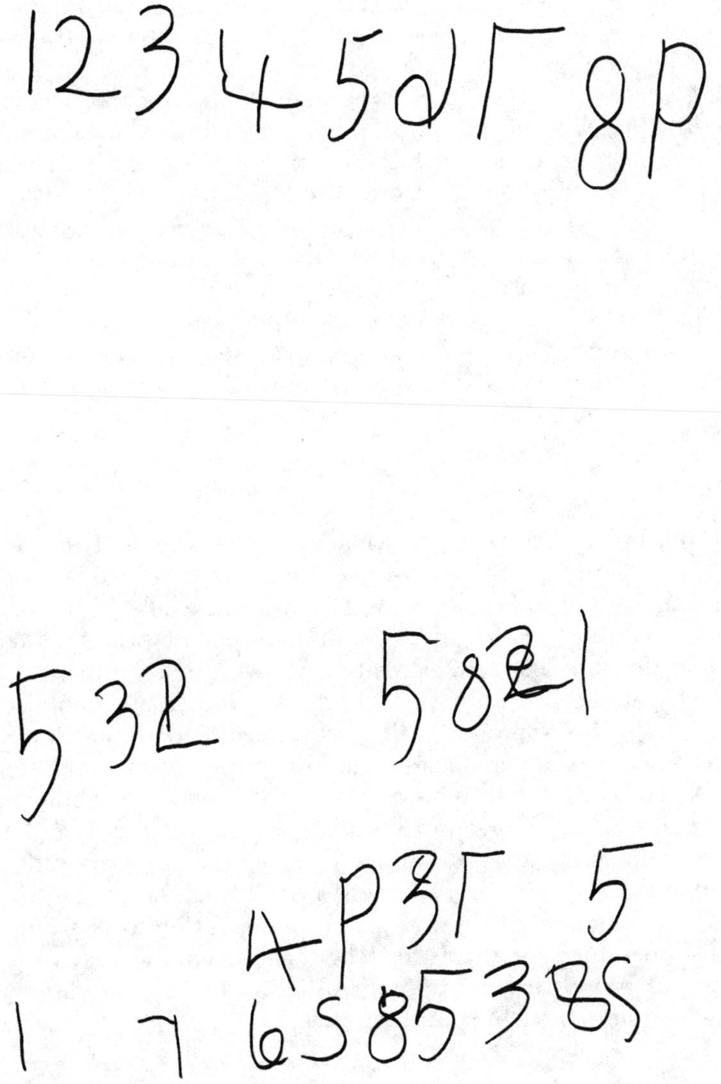

Plate 27. Jason, C.A. 7–8.

Jason's Total VADS Test score of 16 resembled that of 6-year-old children (Appendix B) or end-of-kindergarten pupils (Appendix C). A glance at his four VADS Subtest scores revealed that the Aural-Oral, Visual-Oral, and Aural-Written scores were all within the low average range, whereas the Visual-Written Subtest score fell below the 10th percentile for 7-year-olds (Appendix A). Since the Visual-Oral score, which also involves visual processing was average (25 to 50th percentile), it appeared that Jason did not have difficulty with visual processing as such, but rather that he had specific problems with visual-motor integration. His Written Expression and Intrasensory Integration scores were also very low (below 10th percentile). Jason's Total VADS Test score was at the 10th percentile, whereas the Aural Input, Oral Expression, and Intersensory Integration scores were all low average (25th percentile).

The VADS Test record and his test performance showed that Jason had serious problems with directionality, reversals, sequencing, and with visual-motor integration. He also displayed much immaturity in organization and planning, and an extremely short attention span.

Conclusions

From his VADS Test performance it was apparent that Jason not only looked like an immature 6-year-old child but that he also functioned like one in the area of visual-motor integration and recall. Jason still had much difficulty with the writing of digits; he had specific problems with directionality and digit reversals. Observation showed that Jason was a vulnerable, sensitive youngster with a very short attention span; mental concentration tired him. Yet, his approach to the test reflected good intelligence. Jason was aware of many of his errors and tried to correct them spontaneously.

Jason was a slowly maturing boy. He needed specific help with the organization of his work and with the writing of digits and letters. Jason should be encouraged to verbalize to himself the numbers and words he tries to read and write. He might benefit from visual-motor training. In view of Jason's good mental ability and his high motivation for learning, it appeared that his long-range prognosis for school achievement was good, provided he was permitted to learn and to progress at his own slower rate without undue pressure from his teachers and parents.

2. CASE HISTORY: ANGELO

Angelo was born in Italy. He moved with his family to the United States when he was 3 years old. When he entered kindergarten he knew very little English, since his parents spoke Italian at home. However, Angelo was a very verbal child who learned English quickly, and he was able to express himself in English before long. Yet, the quality of his language remained quite immature, and he failed to make good academic progress in kindergarten and in the first grade. Physically Angelo was tall and well developed, but he acted like a much younger child. He was 7 years 8 months old when his teacher referred him for a psychological evaluation in order to determine whether Angelo's poor language skills and slow academic progress resulted from a culture conflict between his home and school situation, or from other causes.

When I saw Angelo he was friendly, outgoing, chatty, and very cooperative. His speech pattern was quite immature and he had a slight articulation problem. On the WISC-R (Wechsler, 1974) Angelo obtained a Verbal IQ score of 85, a Performance IQ score of 71, and a Full Scale IQ score of 76. Angelo's WISC-R testing age and his Bender Gestalt Test score were at the 6-year-old level. The same was true for his VADS Test performance. Angelo enjoyed the VADS Test and tried hard to do well.

On the *Aural-Oral* Subtest Angelo was able to repeat the three- and four-digit series without error. He then missed both trials on the five-digit series. Angelo was as yet unable to hold and sequence five items of information in his memory. He added, omitted, substituted, and transposed digits as he tried to recall them. *His A-O score was 4.*

On the *Visual-Oral Subtest* Angelo was again only able to repeat the three- and four-digit series. He could not remember more than four digits at a time. He made no attempt to group digits. When the five-digit sequence was presented, the digits either just vanished from his memory or they became all jumbled. *Angelo's V-O score was 4.*

On the *Aural-Written Subtest* Angelo wrote without error the three- and four-digit series. He then lost part of the five-digit sequence on the first trial; on the second trial with a five-digit sequence Angelo recalled all digits correctly, but he transposed the first two digits. *His A-W score was 4.*

On the *Visual-Written Subtest* Angelo was only able to reproduce the three-digit series without error. He neither verbalized the digits nor did he group them to help him with their recall; in consequence, he had difficulty remembering them. On the first four-digit sequence Angelo forgot all but the first digit. On the second four-digit sequence Angelo was able to recall all four digits but he transposed the middle digits. *His V-W score was 3.*

Angelo's VADS Test scores were:

VADS	Score	Percentile	VADS	Score	Percentile
A–O	4	10 to 25	A I	8	10 to 25
V–O	4	10	V I	7	below 10
A–W	4	10 to 25	O E	8	10
V–W	3	below 10	W E	7	below 10
Total	15	below 10	Intra	7	below 10
			Inter	8	10

Angelo was a very verbal youngster and he did relatively better with auditory processing and oral expression than with visual processing and written expression. His overall functioning in integration, sequencing, and recall was below the 10th percentile for 7-year-old pupils (Appendix A). His Total VADS Test score of 15 was on the level of 6-year-old children (Appen-

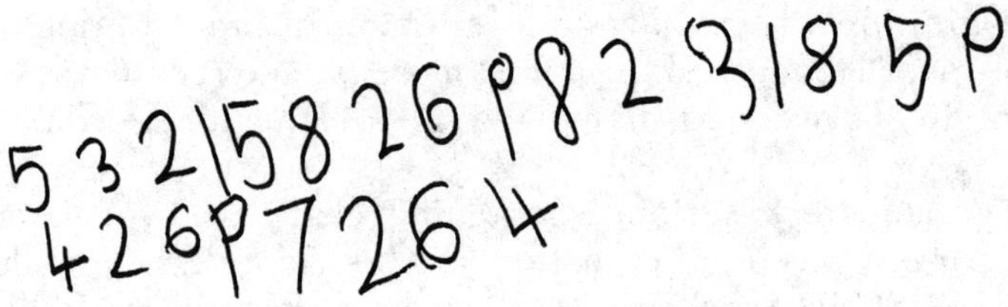

5 3 2 5 8 2 6 8 2 3 8 5

4 2 6 7 2 6 4

Plate 28. Angelo, C.A. 7–8.

dix B) and was typical of average end-of-kindergarten pupils (Appendix C). Angelo's VADS Test scores were in keeping with his test results on the WISC-R and the Bender Gestalt Test.

Angelo's VADS Test record is shown on Plate 28. The arrangement of his digit sequences at the top of the paper in horizontal fashion is quite immature (Table 3) and is consistent with his general level of functioning. Angelo drew a line after the first three digits on the Aural-Written Subtest. This was his only attempt at organizing or structuring the digit sequences on paper. The subsequent digit series were placed one after the other and merged into one another. Angelo's VADS Test record is characteristic of VADS Test records of end-of-kindergarten or beginning first-grade pupils. He still had difficulty with the writing of the digit 9, but his other digits were well formed and correct.

Conclusions

Angelo was a friendly, outgoing 7½-year-old boy of borderline mental ability. His emotional, social, perceptual-motor, and conceptual functioning were all on the level of 6-year-old children. The same was true of his VADS Test scores and of the organization and quality of his VADS Test record. Since Angelo's functioning level was so consistently low it seemed unlikely that he was suffering from any specific problem in integration, sequencing, and recall. It appeared rather that Angelo showed a marked developmental lag and was a somewhat slow youngster.

It was recommended that Angelo be placed in a small transitional class for immature 7- and 8-year-old children where he could be provided with an intensive educational program on the level of beginning first-grade students. He was as yet unable to cope with a second-grade curriculum; since he was tall for his age it seemed unwise to have him repeat the first grade. It was suggested that Angelo be retested with the VADS and the Bender Tests in the middle of the school year to assess his rate of maturation and progress.

3. CASE HISTORY: BRAD

Brad, age 8 years 6 months, was a large, heavyset, sensitive youngster of average mental ability (WISC Full Scale IQ score 98). He had good common sense and was socially mature for his age, but he spoke with a slight slur and had severe learning disabilities. Brad had experienced much teasing at home and in school because of his poor reading and writing ability. Brad was very self-conscious about his academic deficiencies and tried hard to cover them up. He did not want to be singled out for special help; he wanted to be like everyone else. However, Brad was only able to recognize and write a few sight words, and he could add and subtract only numbers from 1 to 9 by counting. Brad had a visual problem and wore glasses. He was astigmatic in both eyes and had poor depth perception that was only partially corrected by his glasses. His parents and teachers attributed Brad's learning difficulties to his visual problems.

When I saw Brad for testing, he was at ease and very cooperative. He worked slowly and deliberately, putting forth much effort.

On the *Aural-Oral Subtest* Brad was unable to repeat more than four digits correctly. He failed both five-digit sequences as a result of omissions and incorrect sequencing of the middle digits of each series. *His A-O score was 4.*

On the *Visual-Oral Subtest* Brad could repeat the four- and five-digit series without error. He missed both six-digit sequences by omitting and transposing some of the middle digits in each series. *His V-O score was 5.*

On the *Aural-Written Subtest* Brad gripped the pencil tightly as he wrote the three- and four-digit series correctly. He wrote slowly and carefully, alternately using his right and left hand for writing. It was apparent that Brad was trying to control his poor fine-motor coordination. On the first five-digit series (96183) Brad omitted the middle digit and wrote 9683, on the second trial with a five-digit series (38159) Brad transposed the middle digits and omitted the last one; he wrote 3851. *His A-W score was 4.*

On the *Visual-Written Subtest* Brad had no difficulty with the three- and four- and five-digit series. He recalled correctly the first and last digits on both trials of the six-digit series but transposed, substituted, and omitted some of the digits in the middle of the sequences. *His V-W score was 5.*

Brad's VADS Test scores were:

VADS	Score	Percentile	VADS	Score	Percentile
A–O	4	10 to 25	A I	8	10
V–O	5	25 to 50	V I	10	25
A–W	4	10 to 25	O E	9	10 to 25
V–W	5	25	W E	9	25
Total	18	17	Intra	9	25
			Inter	9	25

Brad's parents and teachers always assumed that most of his learning problems resulted from his poor vision. The VADS Test scores revealed that Brad had not only some problems with visual processing but that he also showed difficulties with auditory processing and with intersensory integration, sequencing, and recall. His Total VADS Test score of 18 was below the 25th percentile for 8-year-old children (Appendix A). It was on the level of 6½-year-old pupils (Appendix B) or first-graders (Appendix C). His Aural Input score was very poor (10th percentile), whereas all of his other VADS Test scores were within the low average range (25th percentile) for his age level.

The low score in Aural Input was consistent with Brad's WISC scores. His Verbal IQ score of 91 was 15 points lower than his Performance IQ score of 106. Brad scored lowest on the Information, Arithmetic, and Digit Span WISC Subtests, all of which are closely related to auditory processing and recall.

It was noted that most of Brad's errors on the VADS Test consisted of incorrect sequencing or omissions of the middle digits of digit sequences; he

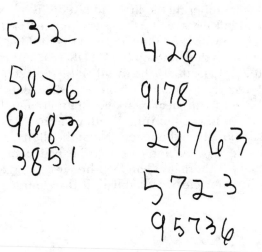

Plate 29. Brad, C.A. 8–6.

usually had no difficulty remembering the first and last digits of a series. The same pattern was observed in Brad's reading and writing; he tended to sound out the first and last letter of a word and then guessed the middle. Brad made no attempt to rehearse or group the digits on the VADS Test and failed to use any sort of learning strategies to facilitate the recall of the digit sequences.

Brad's VADS Test record, as shown on Plate 29, reveals him to be intelligent and a well-controlled, neat worker. Brad arranged the digit sequences in two columns, one for the Aural-Written series and one for the Visual-Written series. The quality and uneven size of the digits, and the way Brad held his pencil while writing, indicate that he had poor fine-motor coordination. The fact that he alternated hands as he wrote suggests that he was ambidextrous and had not clearly established the dominance of one hand over the other.

Conclusions

Brad was a youngster of average mental ability. He had visual problems and wore glasses. His VADS Test performance revealed that he also had problems with auditory processing and with intersensory integration, sequencing, and recall. Brad had poor fine-motor coordination and appeared to be ambidextrous. He was a neat worker and showed good motivation, but he was grossly lacking in learning strategies. On the VADS Test, and when reading, Brad just remembered the first and last letters or digits and then guessed the rest. He needed help with word attack skills, with sequence analysis, and with the grouping and rehearsing of groups of letters and digits. He also needed training to improve his motor coordination and writing skills, and he had to be encouraged to write consistently with one hand. Despite visual problems Brad seemed to learn and recall better what he saw than what he heard.

4. CASE HISTORY: KATHY

Kathy, age 9 years 5 months, was a youngster of average mental ability who functioned academically on the end-of-second-grade level. Kathy was an emotionally and socially deprived child who was starved for attention. She asked if she could go with me and was most cooperative and eager during the testing session. Kathy put forth much effort; her concentration was good although her approach to the VADS Test was immature. She made no attempt to group or to rehearse the digits; she just repeated the digits or wrote them down one by one as they had been presented.

On the *Aural-Oral Subtest* Kathy repeated correctly the four-, five-, and six-digit series. She transposed two digits on both of the seven-digit sequences. *Her A-O score was 6.*

Kathy's performance on the *Visual-Oral Subtest* was near perfect. She recalled the four-, five-, and six-digit series without errors even though she did not group the digits. On the seven-digit series she transposed two digits on the first trial, but reproduced the second seven-digit sequence correctly. *Her V-O score was 7.*

On the *Aural-Written Subtest* Kathy wrote the three- and four-digit series correctly. She missed the first five-digit sequence by transposing the 8 and the 1, but she made no errors on the second five-digit sequences. Kathy missed both trials on the six-digit series as a result of substitutions of the last digits. *Her A-W score was 5.*

On the *Visual-Written Subtest* Kathy showed near perfect visual-motor integration and recall. She had no difficulty with the four- and five-digit series. On the first six-digit sequence Kathy substituted a 6 for a 9 and showed some incorrect sequencing. However, she made no errors on the second six-digit sequence or on the seven-digit series. *Her V-W score was 7.*

Kathy's VADS Test scores were:

VADS	Score	Percentile	VADS	Score	Percentile
A–O	6	50 to 75	A I	11	50
V–O	7	75 to 90	V I	14	75 to 90
A–W	5	50	O E	13	75
V–W	7	75 to 90	W E	12	63
Total	25	75	Intra	13	75
			Inter	12	63

Kathy's VADS Test scores were all in the average to high average range for her age level. Her Total VADS Test score of 25 was at the 75th percentile for 9-year-old children (Appendix A) and resembled the scores of 10-year-old pupils (Appendix B) or average 5th graders (Appendix C). It was apparent that Kathy's intersensory integration, sequencing, and recall were good and that she had above average short-term memory.

Plate 30 shows Kathy's VADS Test record. She wrote with ease, using her right hand. Kathy arranged the digit sequences in a column along the left side of the paper. As she progressed, the lines slanted more and more downward. Halfway through the Visual-Written Subtest, Kathy drew a vertical line alongside the column and began a second column next to the first one, with the remaining digit sequences. The two columns reflect adequate organization and planning ability; however, the vertical line suggests that Kathy had a need for structure and support in order to control her impulsivity (see Chapter 5).

Kathy's good VADS Test scores indicated that her low school achievement did not result from a memory deficit or from problems in intersensory integration, sequencing, and recall. Other factors had to account for her poor reading and arithmetic skills. The only unusual feature of Kathy's VADS Test performance was her failure to use learning strategies (grouping and rehearsing of digits); such a failure is usually found among very young and immature youngsters. A closer look at Kathy's other test results was in order to find additional clues to her poor achievement.

Kathy's WISC-R IQ scores were average (Verbal IQ 98, Performance IQ 101, Full Scale IQ 100). She obtained the highest Verbal Subtest scores in Information, which measures a pupil's long-term memory for facts and figures. On the Performance scale Kathy did best on Picture Completion,

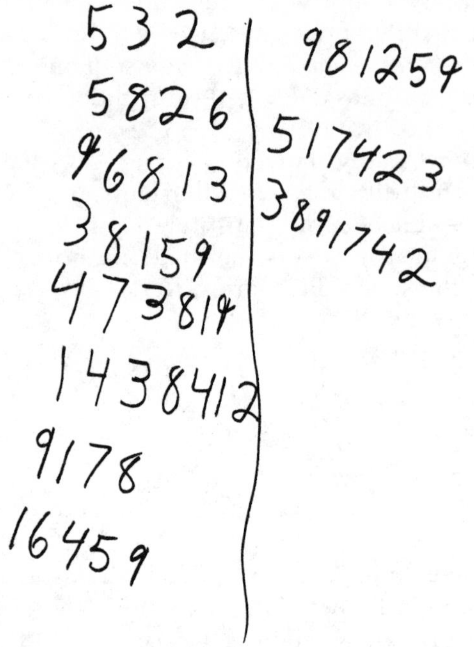

532   981259
5826   517423
46813   3891742
38159
47381 4
1438412
9178
16459

Plate 30. Kathy, C.A. 9–4.

Picture Arrangement, and Object Assembly, all of which deal with pictures and puzzles of concrete objects and situations. The scores on the Subtests involving abstract reasoning (Similarities, Arithmetic, Block Design) were relatively lower. Kathy was a rather concretistic youngster.

On the Wide Range Achievement Test, Kathy displayed serious problems with the discrimination of vowel sounds and with word endings in reading and spelling; she also showed poor understanding of math problems. Kathy worked slowly and with effort and seemed to rely heavily on rote memory. Her word-attack skills were weak, and she was unable to sound out words. In addition, Kathy was handicapped by severe social and emotional impoverishment and by a very unstable family background. She received little stimulation or support for school learning at home. Kathy was a lonely, unhappy youngster with intense feelings of inadequacy.

Conclusions

Kathy was an immature, socially and emotionally deprived, 9½-year-old girl of average mental ability with poor school achievement. On the VADS Test she revealed good concentration, intersensory integration, sequencing, and recall. Her difficulty with schoolwork was evidently not caused by a memory deficit.

Observation and additional test results indicated that Kathy was a somewhat concretistic youngster who had difficulty with the discrimination of vowel sounds and with word endings, with language skills, and with abstract concepts. She used a trial-and-error approach to solving problems, and she relied heavily on rote memory when doing her schoolwork. She received little encouragement or support for school achievement at home, her self-confidence was poor, and she became easily discouraged. All of these factors contributed to Kathy's learning difficulties. In addition, she was a slow and deliberate worker and she did not do well when she was hurried or pressured.

5. CASE HISTORY: TANYA

Tanya, age 10 years 6 months, was referred to the classes for children with learning and behavior disorders because of "major academic and emotional problems." Her behavior was said to vary from cooperative to belligerent. When Tanya was frustrated she screamed, and she had frequent violent fights with her peers. She came from an unstable, socially deprived home background. Her medical record revealed that Tanya had poor auditory acuity for high frequencies, and she was nearsighted and wore glasses. Tanya was of essentially average mental ability (WISC Verbal IQ 87, Performance IQ 97, Full Scale IQ 91) but was unable to read or write more than a few sight words, and she could only add and subtract by counting. When I administered the VADS Test to Tanya she was at ease and highly motivated to do well on the test. Her VADS Test performance was most unusual.

On the *Aural-Oral Subtest* Tanya was only able to repeat the four-digit series. She made sequencing errors and substituted and omitted the last digits on both the five-digit series. *Her A-O score was 4.*

On the *Visual-Oral Subtest* Tanya was only able to repeat the four-digit and five-digit series correctly, she missed both of the six-digit series as a result of errors in sequencing and substitution of the last two digits, even though she organized and grouped the digits by twos. *Her V-O score was 5.*

On the *Aural-Written Subtest* Tanya traced the digits with her finger in the air as she listened to them. She then wrote them with her right hand, holding the pencil awkwardly. Tanya's fine-motor control was poor. She wrote the three-digit sequence (532) vertically and underlined it, and then wrote the four-digit series (5826) horizontally. Both sequences were correct. On the first trial of the five-digit series Tanya was distracted and was only able to produce a 9; the rest escaped her. On the second five-digit series (38159) Tanya reproduced the digits correctly but in the last moment she changed the last two digits and transposed them. *Her A-W score was 4.*

On the *Visual-Written Subtest* Tanya grouped the digits by twos as she said them to herself while writing. Once again she wrote the three-digit series (426) vertically, and corrected the last digit from a 4 to a 6. She then wrote the four-, five-, and six-digit series without errors horizontally. On the first trial with a seven-digit series Tanya recalled the first five digits correctly then added 23 instead of 42. On the second trial she was able to write the seven-digit sequence (7964835) without errors. *Her V-W score was 7.*

Tanya's VADS Test scores were:

VADS	Score	Percentile	VADS	Score	Percentile
A–O	4	below 10	A I	8	below 10
V–O	5	10	V I	12	25
A–W	4	10	O E	9	below 10
V–W	7	50 to 90	W E	11	25
Total	20	10	Intra	11	25
			Inter	9	10

Tanya showed serious deficits in auditory processing (A I), oral expression (OE), and in oral-visual and visual-oral integration (Intersensory Integration). Her Total VADS Test score of 20 was at the 10th percentile for 10-year-old children (Appendix A) and resembled the scores of 7½-year-old pupils (Appendix B) or second-graders (Appendix C).

Tanya's VADS Test record shown on Plate 31 was of particular interest. It reflected her impulsivity, poor organization, and lack of control. The record is characteristic of acting-out youngsters and corresponded to Tanya's actual behavior in school. The line she drew under the first series of digits suggests a need and desire for structure and outer control since her inner control and organization were so weak (see p. 47).

Despite Tanya's disorganized VADS Test record and her poor VADS Test scores, she also revealed signs of intelligence and an effort to compensate for her difficulties (see p. 21). She traced the auditorily presented digits with her finger in the air to help her recall them, and she grouped and rehearsed the visually presented digits.

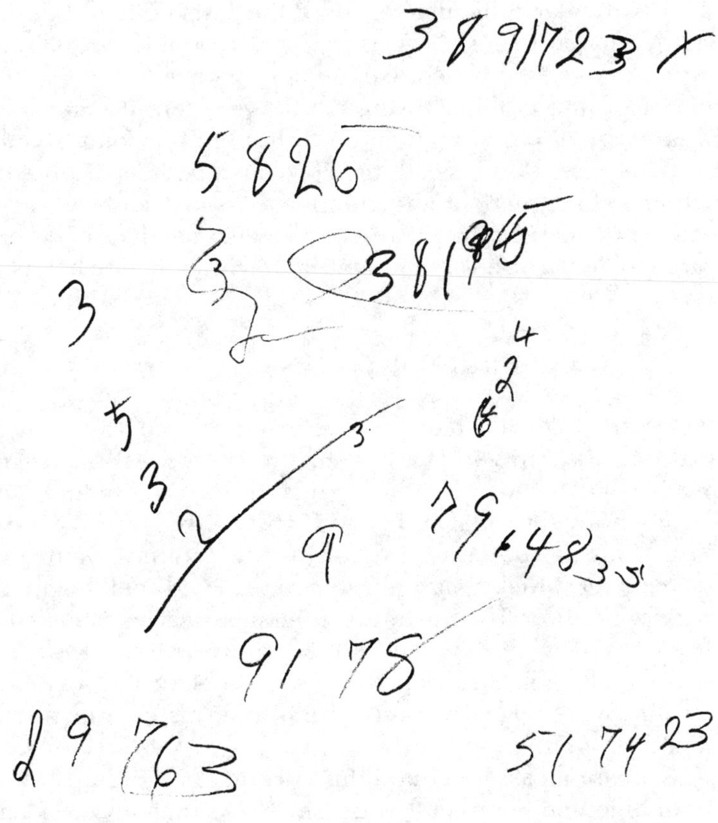

3 8 91723 Y

5826

381 95

3

3

5
3
3

3

9

4
2
6

79 4835

91 78

29 763

51 74 23

Plate 31. Tanya, C.A. 10–6.

Conclusions

Tanya's performance on the VADS Test showed her to be an impulsive, disorganized, acting-out youngster of normal mental ability with poor inner control. She needed outer control and much structure in order to be able to function in school. Tanya suffered from a severe deficit in aural processing, oral expression, and intersensory integration, sequencing, and recall. It was noted that she had particular difficulty recalling the last digits of the digit series and the last letters on words she was trying to read and write. Tanya also dropped word endings when she talked.

Tanya's severe learning problems were to a large extent the result of a hearing loss and language problems, and a disability to form sound-symbol associations and to sequence and recall symbol constellations. Tanya had difficulties following oral instructions and group discussions, and had severe problems remembering what she had learned. She also needed much help with the organization of her written assignments and with her work habits.

6. CASE HISTORY: RICKY

Ricky, age 10 years 1 month, had been referred to a special class for children with learning disabilities. He was an immature, restless, highly distractible youngster with a short attention span and serious problems with visual fusion. Despite normal mental ability (WISC-R Verbal IQ 101, Performance IQ 92, Full Scale IQ 96) and years of private tutoring, optometric training, and special glasses, Ricky was only able to read and spell beginning second-grade words with effort. His frustration tolerance was low and he had become quite discouraged when he could not keep up with his peers in a regular fourth grade. Ricky adjusted well to the special class and was much relieved that he could work without undue pressure at his own level with much individualized support.

When I saw Ricky for an assessment of his current level of functioning, he was very cooperative and completely at ease. He volunteered, "I have exactly the same kind of problems with my eyes as the vice-president of the United States (Rockefeller), that is why I need more time to learn to read." Ricky was confident that in good time he too would be able to read. His emotional and social adjustment was fairly good.

Ricky's approach to the VADS Test showed good intelligence as well as much impulsivity. He worked very rapidly and needed frequent reminders to slow down and to look at the test cards as long as they were shown to him. Ricky verbalized and rehearsed the digits as he heard or read them; he reorganized them and grouped them by twos and threes.

On the *Aural-Oral Subtest* Ricky repeated the four-digit series correctly, but missed the first trial with the five-digit series as a result of a minor sequencing error. Ricky recalled the second five-digit sequence and the six-digit series without errors. He failed both trials with the seven-digit sequences, showing mainly transposition or sequencing mistakes. *His A-O score was 6.*

On the *Visual-Oral Subtest* Ricky had no difficulty with the four- and five-digit series. Sequencing errors were again evident on both trials with the six-digit series. *His V-O score was 5.*

On the *Aural-Written Subtest* Ricky wrote the four-digit sequence correctly but reversed the 5. On the first five-digit sequence he transposed two digits and reversed a 3. Ricky reproduced the second five-digit sequence without errors, although he again reversed the 5. He failed both trials with the six-digit series because of errors in sequencing, substitutions, and omissions of digits. *His A-W score was 5.*

On the *Visual-Written Subtest* Ricky wrote correctly the four-, five-, and six-digit sequences. He missed the first seven-digit sequence by omitting one digit. Unfortunately time did not permit the administration of the second trial with the seven-digit series, since Ricky had to go to another class. But it is questionable whether he would have been able to pass the second trial since he was getting visibly tired and restless. Sustained mental concentration was difficult for him, even though his motivation for achievement was good. *His V-W score was 6.*

Ricky's VADS Test scores were:

VADS	Score	Percentile	VADS	Score	Percentile
A–O	6	50	A I	11	38
V–O	5	10	V I	11	10
A–W	5	25 to 50	O E	11	25
V–W	6	25	W E	11	25
Total	22	25	Intra	12	38
			Inter	10	25

The VADS Test scores show that auditory processing was easier for Ricky than was visual processing. His Aural Input score was at the 38th percentile for 10-year-olds, whereas his Visual Input score was at the 10th percentile. Ricky had particular problems with visual-oral integration, sequencing, and recall. Visual processing and visual-oral integration are, of course, most closely related to school achievement (Chapter 11). Ricky's Total VADS Test score of 22 was at the 25th percentile for 10-year-old children (Appendix A) and resembled the scores of average 8½ year olds (Appendix B) or third-grade pupils (Appendix C).

Ricky's VADS Test record is shown on Plate 32. The digit sequences were well organized into a single column. The rather poor formation of the individual digits reflected Ricky's impulsivity, poor fine-motor coordination, and the haste with which they were written. Most outstanding are the reversals of two of the 5s and 3s. Reversals are most unusual on the VADS Test records of 10-year-old-children of normal intelligence; they indicate serious problems with directionality.

Conclusions

Ricky was a cheerful, restless, immature 10-year-old boy of normal mental ability who had serious learning problems. His VADS Test performance showed much impulsivity and a short attention span. He had severe problems with visual processing and with visual-oral integration and recall.

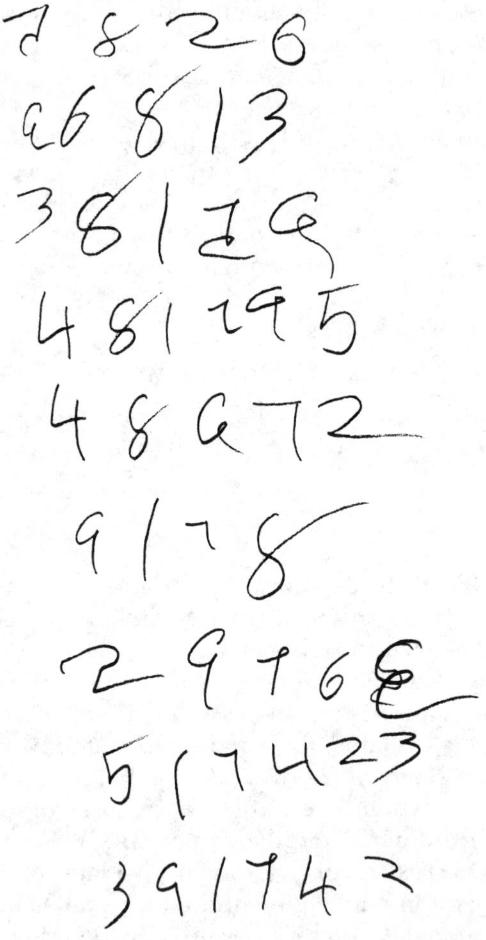

7 8 2 6
6 6 8 1 3
3 8 1 2 6
4 8 1 2 9 5
4 8 6 7 2
9 1 7 8
2 9 7 6 6
5 1 7 4 2 3
3 9 1 7 4 3

Plate 32. Ricky, C.A. 10–1.

Ricky's fine-motor coordination was poor, and he exhibited particular difficulties with directionality and with the sequencing of digits. Ricky and his
parents blamed his learning disabilities entirely on his problems with visual
fusion, but the VADS Test revealed that very poor intersensory integration
and recall also contributed greatly to Ricky's reading and writing disabilities.
He was able to see digits correctly, but when he wrote digits he could not
automatically remember whether they faced to the right or to the left, nor
could he recall the symbol or sound sequences when he tried to reproduce
what he had heard or seen.

Ricky's approach to the VADS Test reflected good mental ability; he
used verbal rehearsal and grouping of digits to help him remember them
better. However, he worked too rapidly for these strategies to be effective
and his writing was sloppy. It was recommended that Ricky be taught to slow
down, to improve his writing skills, and to check on himself for digit and
letter reversals. Since Ricky seemed to be an auditory learner, he needed to
be encouraged to vocalize to himself when trying to learn visual material. He
needed specific training in dealing with directions and sequences.

7. CASE HISTORY: DON

Don, age 11 years 5 months, was a friendly, immature, neurologically
impaired youngster who had attended special classes for children with
learning disabilities since he was 7 years old. Don had difficulty coping with
group situations; his relationships with peers were very poor. He was bothered by loud noises , and he was rigid and became upset when there was any
sudden or unexpected change in his routine. In school he was a loner and
spent most of the time at his desk either working or "resting." Don's
achievement in reading, spelling, and arithmetic was at the fourth-grade
level. He was grossly lacking in common-sense reasoning and functioned
quite unevenly. On the WISC-R, Don obtained a Verbal IQ score of 87, a
Performance IQ score of 58, and a Full Scale IQ score of 71.

When I administered the VADS Test to Don he was at ease and enjoyed
the attention he received. Don repeated and wrote the digits one by one just
as they were presented; he made no attempt to group or to rehearse the digits
in order to facilitate their recall. Don was pleased with his achievement on
the VADS Test and congratulated himself. He showed all the self-centered-
ness and naiveté of a much younger child.

On the *Aural-Oral Subtest* Don repeated the four-, five-, and six-digit
series without errors. On the seven-digit series Don recalled all of the digits
correctly but transposed two digits on each of the two trials. *His A-O score
was 6.*

On the *Visual-Oral Subtest* Don recalled correctly the five-, six-, and
seven-digit series. *His V-O score was 7.*

On the *Aural-Written Subtest* Don wrote with ease the four-, five-, and
six-digit series without errors. He then repeated all of the digits in the seven-
digit series correctly but made minor sequencing errors on both trials. *His
A-W score was 6.*

On the *Visual-Written Subtest* Don failed both trials with the five-digit series as a result of errors in sequencing and substitutions. I thereupon gave Don a four-digit sequence that he reproduced correctly. Don wrote the visually presented digits without translating them into auditory patterns and saying them to himself or rehearsing them. He relied entirely on his visual memory. *His V-W score was 4.*

Don's VADS Test scores were:

VADS	Score	Percentile	VADS	Score	Percentile
A–O	6	50	A I	12	50
V–O	7	50 to 90	V I	11	10
A–W	6	50	O E	13	50
V–W	4	below 10	W E	10	10
Total	23	25	Intra	10	below 10
			Inter	13	50

Don's Aural-Oral, Visual-Oral, and Aural-Written Subtest scores were all average, whereas his Visual-Written Subtest score was quite defective, falling below the 10th percentile for his age level. It appears that Don had a specific problem with visual-motor integration and recall (see p. 124). Despite the low score on Visual Input, it was clear that Don did not have difficulties with visual perception or visual processing since his Visual-Oral Subtest score was high average. And despite the very low score on Written Expression, Don did not have serious problems with writing since his Aural-Written score was average. The Visual-Written Subtest differs from the other three Subtests in that it does not explicitly involve language. Children who do well on the Visual-Written Subtest spontaneously translate the visually presented digits into language; they say the digits to themselves, either vocally or subvocally. Most youngsters also group and rehearse the digits as a means of recalling them better. Don did none of this. He was too rigid and concretistic to do anything other than what he was specifically told to do. Extreme rigidity was also reflected in Don's very low score (below 10th percentile) in Intrasensory Integration (see p. 134). Don lacked the initiative to develop learning strategies on his own.

Don's poor Visual-Written Subtest score was consistent with his very immature performance on the Bender Gestalt Test and with his defective WISC Performance IQ score. He suffered from severe problems in visual-motor integration. Don's Total VADS Test score of 23 was low average or in the 25th percentile for 11-year-old children (Appendix A). The score was typical of average 9-year-old children (Appendix B) and of fourth-grade pupils (Appendix C).

Don's VADS Test record, as shown on Plate 33, reflected good organization and work habits. He arranged the digit sequences into two neat columns placed beneath each other. The unevenness in the size of the digits indicated some weakness in motor coordination.

Conclusions

Don's VADS Test performance showed that he was a youngster with much unevenness in functioning. His auditory processing and visual-oral

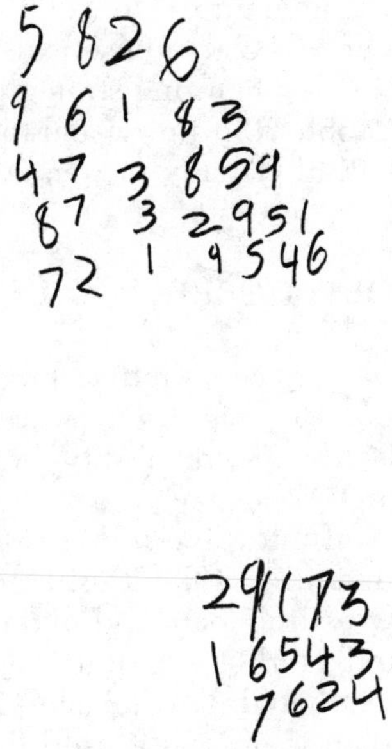

5 8 2 6
9 6 1 8 3
4 7 3 8 5 9
8 7 3 2 9 5 1
7 2 1 9 5 4 6

2 9 1 7 3
1 6 5 4 3
7 6 2 4

Plate 33. Don, C.A. 11–5.

recall were quite good, whereas his visual-motor integration was extremely poor and his fine-motor coordination was immature. Don, age 11½, was very rigid and concretistic; he lacked initiative and common sense reasoning, and needed explicit directions on how to develop learning strategies and how to solve a problem. Don had a specific problem in the visual-motor area and needed help with the copying and recall of visually presented material.

8. CASE HISTORY: HERBIE

Herbie, age 11 years 9 months, was very cooperative during the testing session. Herbie always loved attention. He was a good-natured, restless, impulsive, talkative youngster of borderline mental ability (WISC-R Verbal IQ 72, Performance IQ 68, Full Scale IQ 68) who was still a nonreader, despite good motivation and five years of intensive individualized help in small special classes for children with learning difficulties. Herbie achieved his greatest successes on the school's wrestling team and in the drum corps.

When the VADS Test was presented, Herbie was quite enthusiastic and worked very rapidly. Since he was a rather dull youngster I began each Subtest with a lower series of digits than is normally used for 11-year-old children (see p. 13).

On the *Aural-Oral Subtest* Herbie repeated the four-, five-, and six-digit series correctly, then missed both seven-digit series as a result of errors in sequencing. *His A-O score was 6.*

On the *Visual-Oral Subtest* Herbie repeated correctly the four-digit series. After missing the first five-digit series, he reproduced the second five-digit series without error. Then he failed both six-digit series as a result of sequencing errors and the omission of a digit. *His V-O score was 5.*

On the *Aural-Written Subtest* Herbie had no difficulty with the three- and four-digit series. But as can be seen on Plate 34 he had considerable problems with the five-digit series. Herbie verbalized the digits "96183" correctly as he wrote 981, interchanging the 8 for the 6; he was aware that something was wrong and hesitated, then continued to write 123. This time he substituted the 2 for the 8. Although Herbie knew that his response was not right, he could not correct it since he had forgotten the sequence of digits in the meantime.

I thereupon gave Herbie the second five-digit series that he repeated without error orally, but when he tried to write the sequence down he omitted the 5, thus writing 3819 instead of 38159. Once again Herbie was aware of his mistake; this time he even recalled that a 5 was missing, however, he did not remember where the 5 belonged and placed it at the beginning of the series. Since he came so close to writing a correct sequence I gave Herbie a chance to recall a six-digit series (473859). Herbie began by *writing 45* even though he *said 47.* Realizing his error he crossed out the 45 and began over again, writing correctly 4738. This time he omitted the 5 altogether and completed the series with a 9. *His A-W score was 4.*

On the *Visual-Written Subtest* Herbie refused to wait 10 seconds before

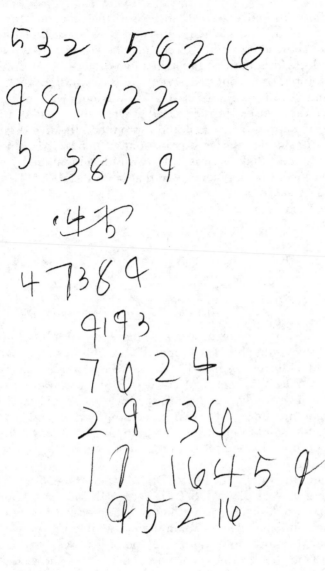

Plate 34. Herbie, C.A. 11–9.

starting to write the digits. In consequence, he missed the first four-digit series, writing 9193 instead of 9178. When I insisted that he look at the stimulus card as long as I showed it to him (10 seconds), he was able to write the second four-digit series without error. On the first five-digit series Herbie *said* the digits in their proper order but transposed the last two digits as he *wrote* them, thus writing 29736 instead of 29763. He was not aware of his error. On the second five-digit series Herbie started to write 19 instead of 16 but he caught himself. He started over again and reproduced the five-digit series correctly. When the six-digit series was presented (985216), Herbie omitted the 8. He announced that he was getting tired, and indeed he seemed to be unable to concentrate any longer. At that point the VADS Test was discontinued. *His V-W score was 5.*

Herbie's VADS Test scores were:

VADS	Score	Percentile	VADS	Score	Percentile
A–O	6	50	A I	10	18
V–O	5	10	V I	10	below 10
A–W	4	10	O E	11	18
V–W	5	10	W E	9	below 10
Total	20	below 10	Intra	11	10
			Inter	9	below 10

Herbie's Total VADS Test score of 20 was extremely low; it fell below the 10th percentile for 11-year-old children (Appendix A). The score was on the level of 7½-year-old children (Appendix B) or second-grade pupils (Appendix C). Herbie's VADS Test score pattern was very immature; only the Aural-Oral Subtest score was average for his age level (see p. 119). He suffered from serious malfunctioning in visual processing, written expression, intrasensory integration, and intersensory integration. Herbie did relatively better (18th percentile) with aural processing and oral expression since he was a very verbal youngster.

Herbie's behavior and the quality of his VADS Test performance were diagnostically as revealing as were his VADS Test scores. He was extremely impulsive and dashed into the task at hand without waiting for instructions. He never stopped to look and analyze a problem before giving a response. When Herbie was made to slow down and wait before answering, his performance improved. Thus, one of the major efforts in class was directed toward getting Herbie to work more slowly and to stop and think before acting.

Herbie revealed serious problems with sequencing and with written expression. He repeatedly *wrote* the wrong digits even while *saying* them correctly. He needed help with listening to his own verbal instructions, and with checking his written work since he could not depend on what he put down on paper.

Like many dull youngsters, Herbie showed a marked weakness in developing and using learning strategies and in the organization of his work. He failed to group or to rehearse digits as he repeated them and wrote them. He also made no attempt to erase or correct incorrect digits; instead he crossed them out impulsively and wrote the digits over again. Herbie required specific instructions on how to organize and structure the material he was trying to learn and to remember.

Herbie had a short attention span and tired quickly. Since he was poorly integrated, any mental concentration was difficult for him; it demanded an exorbitant amount of energy on his part. In class Herbie was only able to cope with brief assignments and needed a frequent change of pace and activities.

Conclusions

Herbie was an 11½-year-old boy of borderline mental ability. His VADS Test performance showed him to be a very impulsive, poorly integrated, immature youngster with a short attention span, poor sequencing and recall, and limited reasoning ability; he had specific problems in visual-motor integration, visual processing, and written expression. All of this grossly interfered with his academic progress. He learned best in a highly structured situation when he was given oral instructions and could give verbal responses. Herbie had to learn to take time out to check on his written work since he frequently wrote incorrect answers even when he knew the correct answers. Above all Herbie needed to slow down and to control his impulsivity and restlessness.

9. CASE HISTORY: TODD

Todd, age 12 years 4 months, had been placed into a special sixth-grade core class for children with limited mental ability. He had a long history of poor school achievement and had repeated the first grade. Todd was small for his age, timid, and unable to complete his assignments, yet, he seemed alert and showed a keen interest in science. His teacher questioned whether Todd was truly a slow child and referred him for psychological evaluation.

When I saw Todd he was friendly, outgoing, and quite chatty; he tried to please the examiner. On the WISC-R, Todd obtained a Verbal IQ score of 107, a Performance IQ score of 111, and a Full Scale IQ score of 110. Todd did particularly well on the tests of verbal and visual abstract reasoning; his test scores were 13 for Similarities, 14 for Vocabulary, and 12 for Block Design. The teacher's observations had been correct. Obviously Todd was a youngster of high average mental ability, but he had serious specific learning disabilities. His reading, spelling, and arithmetic skills, as measured on the Wide Range Achievement Test, were only at the beginning fourth-grade level.

The VADS Test proved to be of great diagnostic value. Todd worked very slowly and deliberately; nothing was easy or automatic for him. He put forth much effort and showed good intelligence in his approach to the test. Todd grouped the digits by twos and threes, rehearsed them verbally as he tried to remember them, and traced digits with his finger in the air.

On the *Aural-Oral Subtest* Todd was able to repeat without errors the five- and six-digit series, but he missed both seven-digit sequences as a result of his difficulty with the sequencing of the last three digits of the series. *His A-O score was 6.*

On the *Visual-Oral Subtest,* Todd missed the first five-digit sequence when he transposed the third and fourth digits, but he repeated the second five-digit sequence without error. Todd failed both six-digit series, and showed errors in sequencing and omissions. *His V-O score was 5.*

On the *Aural-Written Subtest* Todd reproduced correctly the three- and four-digit series. On the first trial with the five-digit series he transposed the third and fourth digits. On the second trial with the five-digit series Todd substituted a 3 for the 9 at the end of the series. *His A-W score was 4.*

On the Visual-Written Subtest Todd wrote the four-, five-, and six-digit series without errors, but then he showed sequencing errors on both trials with the seven-digit series. *His V-W score was 6.*

Todd's VADS Test scores were:

VADS	Score	Percentile	VADS	Score	Percentile
A–O	6	25 to 50	A I	10	10
V–O	5	10	V I	11	below 10
A–W	4	below 10	O E	11	10
V–W	6	10	W E	10	below 10
Total	21	below 10	Intra	12	25
			Inter	9	below 10

Only the Aural-Oral and Intrasensory Integration scores were within the average range of VADS Test scores for 12-year-old children. Todd had serious problems with visual and auditory processing, sequencing, intersensory integration, and recall. His Total VADS Test score of 21 fell below the 10th percentile for his age level (Appendix A) and resembled the average scores of 8-year-old youngsters (Appendix B) or second-grade pupils (Appendix C).

The problems revealed on the VADS Test were closely related to Todd's school achievement. In reading, Todd was able to sound out each individual letter, but he had great difficulty integrating and sequencing the letters and sounds. His sight vocabulary was quite limited since his visual memory was poor. Todd had particular difficulty with word endings just as he had most problems with the recall of the last few digits on the digit sequences.

In Plate 35, which shows Todd's VADS Test record, it can be seen that he arranged the digit sequences neatly along the edge of the paper; Todd needed structure and support since his inner control was weak (see p. 47). Todd worked very slowly and wrote the digits with great care. He required an unusually long time to complete the VADS Test since he had to consciously compensate for his poor integration and recall. He was unable to work fast, and it was apparent that Todd could not possibly complete his class assignments in the time usually allotted by teachers. When he was pushed or pressured, Todd could not concentrate and gave up; he withdrew and just sat and did nothing.

532
5826
96813
38153
9178
29763
985216
389721
5832156

Plate 35. Todd, C.A. 12–4.

Conclusions

Todd was an immature 12½-year-old boy of high average mental ability; his reasoning ability was good but he had serious specific learning difficulties. His VADS Test performance showed that he suffered from severe problems in auditory and visual processing, sequencing, intersensory integration, and recall, all of which contributed to his low academic achievement. Todd had particular problems in reading and spelling since his poor visual memory interfered with the acquisition of a good sight vocabulary. He failed to benefit from a phonetic approach to reading, since he had difficulty in forming symbol-sound associations and blending sounds because of his problems with sequencing and intersensory integration.

Todd's VADS Test scores were on the level of 8-year-old children. His approach to the test revealed good intelligence; he spontaneously used learning strategies (grouping, rehearsing, tracing of digits) and organized his VADS Test record well. Todd needed structure and control and could only work if he was given much time. He worked very slowly and deliberately since he had to compensate for his learning disabilities. Todd was obviously not a mentally slow child but he did need special help. Todd was transferred to a regular 6th-grade class and each day was given two periods of intensive help and support in the school's Resource Room.

10. CASE HISTORY: ANNA

Anna, age 12 years 5 months, had recently moved into the school district. She seemed overwhelmed by the large new middle school and was unable to cope with any of the academic subjects. In class, Anna sat quietly at her desk working, but she showed very little understanding of what she was doing. Between classes, Anna raced down the halls and frequently got involved in fights with both boys and girls. Anna was physically well developed, but she was grossly lacking in social judgment. She was referred by her teachers for psychological evaluation to assess her mental ability and to help plan an educational program for her.

Anna obtained a WISC-R Verbal IQ score of 67, a Performance IQ score of 65, and a Full Scale IQ score of 64. She was a moderately retarded youngster with a testing age of 8. All of Anna's WISC-R Subtest scores were low; there was little intertest scatter. Her highest Subtest score was a 7 on the Digit Span Test. Anna had evidently fairly adequate recall and visual recognition. She was able to read and spell fourth-grade words, even though she could only read third-grade books with comprehension. When I administered the VADS Test, Anna was most cooperative and put forth effort.

On the *Aural-Oral Subtest* Anna repeated the five- and six-digit series without errors; she then missed both seven-digit sequences as a result of an omission of the last digits. *Her A-O score was 6.*

On the *Visual-Oral Subtest* Anna correctly recalled the five- and six-digit series. She missed the first seven-digit sequence by omitting one digit, but repeated the second seven-digit sequence without error. *Her V-O score was 7.*

On the *Aural-Written Subtest* Anna reproduced correctly the four-, five-, and six-digit series. She missed both trials with the seven-digit series as a result of omissions and sequencing errors. *Her A-W score was 6.*

On the *Visual-Written Subtest* Anna wrote the four-, five-, six-, and seven-digit series without errors. *Her V-W score was 7.*

Anna's VADS Test scores were:

VADS	Score	Percentile	VADS	Score	Percentile
A–O	6	25 to 50	A I	12	50
V–O	7	50 to 90	V I	14	50 to 90
A–W	6	50	O E	13	50
V–W	7	25 to 90	W E	13	50
Total	26	50	Intra	13	50
			Inter	13	50

All of Anna's VADS Test scores were within the average range for 12-year-old children; that is, Anna's VADS Test performance was appropriate for her age level (Appendix A) despite her limited mental ability. Most retarded youngsters have difficulty with sequencing and recall (see p. 113), but there are exceptions (Spitz, 1973). Anna was one of them. Her memory was average, and she learned mainly by rote.

Of particular interest was Anna's VADS Test record, which is shown on Plate 36. Anna gave herself guidelines and imposed a structure on the blank piece of paper. She had been apparently trained to do this and did it effectively. Her work habits were excellent. Before Anna started to write a digit series she numbered the response and drew a line, and then placed the digit sequence on the line. Anna needed structure and outer control in order to function in school. Without such structure Anna became disorganized and yielded to her impulses. This was clearly demonstrated in her performance on the less structured Bender Gestalt Test. She showed a lack of planning and spread the nine Bender Test designs over two sheets of paper, which is most unusual for 12-year-old pupils. Her Bender Test protocol showed a great deal of disorganization and impulsivity and was typical of the Bender Test records of many aggressive and acting-out youngsters.

The same type of discrepancy that was shown between the well-organized record of the more structured VADS Test and the highly disorganized protocol of the less structured Bender Test was also evident in Anna's behavior in school. In the structured classroom, under the watchful eye of her teacher, Anna was well behaved and worked diligently even when she did not understand the work, but in the less structured school halls and cafeteria Anna roamed about and displayed much impulsivity and aggressive behavior. Anna's case illustrates how neither the VADS Test nor the Bender Gestalt Test alone provided a rounded picture of the child's functioning. But together they revealed valuable information and showed how essential it was that Anna be provided with a highly structured, special school program.

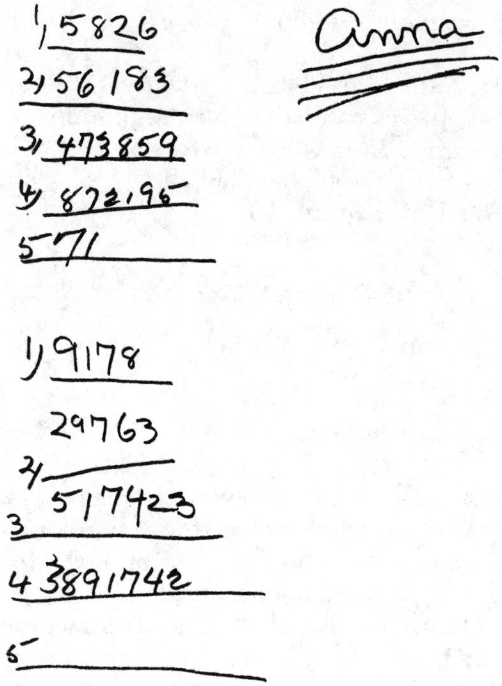

1, 5826   *anna*

3, 56183

3, 473859

4, 872195

5, 71

1) 9178

2, 9763

2,

3   517423

4 3891742

5

Plate 36. Anna, C.A. 12–5.

Conclusions

Anna was a moderately retarded, impulsive 12½-year-old girl who func-tioned quite low in all areas, with the exception of visual recognition and short-term memory. Anna's performance on the VADS Test was average for her age level; the VADS Test revealed her area of strength. Anna had fairly good reading recognition and spelling ability. She learned mainly by rote, but her comprehension was very poor.

Anna showed good work habits and was a willing student as long as she was in a highly structured and supportive classroom setting. In a less structured situation she followed her impulses, became disorganized, and got into fights with peers. She lacked common sense and social judgment. The VADS Test as well as the Bender Gestalt Test each reflected one of these conflicting aspects of Anna's behavior. Together the VADS Test and the Bender Test gave a rounded picture and showed Anna's need for structure and support and her ability to learn by rote and to work well when she was given explicit directions and outer controls.

Chapter 15

The VADS Test as Part of a Screening
Battery for School Beginners

The preceding case histories demonstrated that the VADS Test is a versatile clinical instrument in its own right. But the VADS Test is even more meaningful when it is interpreted together with the results from other psychological tests. This is particularly true when the VADS Test is used as a screening test for school beginners. School achievement depends on many different factors, not all of which are reflected on the VADS Test performance of schoolchildren.

It was shown previously that the VADS Test and the Bender Gestalt Test are both related to achievement and to learning difficulties, but they revealed little relationship to each other. The VADS Test and the Bender Test were found to supplement each other as diagnostic and screening instruments. The VADS Test assesses intersensory integration, sequencing, and recall, and correlates well with reading, spelling, and arithmetic, whereas the Bender Gestalt Test measures visual-motor perception and is most closely related to overall school functioning and mental ability. The test records of both the Bender Test and the VADS Test can be analyzed for organization and planning ability, for fine-motor coordination, and for impulsivity and acting-out tendencies. But even these two tests together are not sufficient to evaluate school beginners for potential learning difficulties. Children's functioning in school is also greatly influenced by their social and emotional adjustment. The Human Figure Drawing Test (hereafter HFD) was shown to be especially valuable in assessing this factor, as well as mental maturity (Koppitz, 1968).

Based on my research and experience, I have found that the VADS Test, the Bender Test, and the HFD together form a useful screening battery for end-of-kindergarten and beginning first-grade pupils. This battery is brief and effective. The Bender Test and HFDs can be administered individually or as group tests to school beginners (Koppitz, 1975a, p. 109 ff), whereas the VADS Test has to be administered individually to each youngster. The group administration saves time, but it is important to give at least one short individual test so as to provide the examiner with the opportunity to observe the child at work and obtain a sample of his speech and language ability.

The screening battery for school beginners and its application has been described and illustrated in detail in the *Bender Gestalt Test for young children, Volume II, Research and application, 1963–1973* (Koppitz, 1975a, p. 99–108). Three examples are presented here to demonstrate how the

Bender Test, the VADS Test, and the HFDs each can reveal different areas of strength or weakness in end-of-kindergarten pupils that the other two tests fail to identify.

The youngsters' performance on the screening battery is analyzed for the developmental scores, for the quality of the test records, and for Emotional Indicators. Table 31 shows the interpretation of the developmental scores of all three tests and of the number of reversals on the VADS Test. The Bender Test was analyzed for Developmental scores and for Emotional Indicators (Koppitz, 1975a, Table 15 and pp. 83 ff); the VADS Test score levels were taken from Appendix C, whereas the number of digit reversals came from Table 2. A detailed description of the Developmental scores and the Emotional Indicators on the HFDs can be found in *Psychological Evaluation of Children's Human Figure Drawings* (Koppitz, 1968).

All of the information gathered from the three test records is recorded and summarized on a *Screening Battery Summary Sheet*. There is no hard and fast formula that can be applied to the interpretation of the test scores and other data. I am opposed to combining scores from different tests into a single score with a cutoff point for the prediction of school success or failure. A meaningful prediction of a child's potential for school achievement and for possible learning problems has to involve a careful assessment and integration of different kinds of information and should not be based on single test scores. The use of the screening battery is simple, but it does require training and experience in the use of the Bender Test, the VADS Test, and the HFDs. In the hands of a qualified and skilled examiner the three tests together can be most helpful in pinpointing areas of strength and weakness in a child, for suggesting ways to develop individualized educational programs to meet the youngster's needs, and for planning the pupil's class placement. The results of the screening battery should be discussed with the classroom teacher. Any plans for a child's educational program and placement has to result, of course, from a combination of the teacher's recommendations, the findings of the screening battery, and a discussion with the pupil's parents.

The youngsters used in the following three examples were part of an entire kindergarten class to whom I gave the screening battery at the end of the school year. I administered the Bender Test, the VADS Test, and the HFD to each child individually in the back of the classroom. I asked each

Table 31.

Interpretation of Test Scores for End-of-Kindergarten Pupils

Level of Test Scores	Bender Test Score	Total VADS Test Scores	Reversals on VADS Test	Developmental Score on HFD
Outstanding	5 or less	19 or more	0	6 or more
High	6 or 7	17 or 18	1	5 or 6
Average	8 to 11	13 to 16	2 or 3	4 or 5
Low	12 or 13	11 or 12	4	3
Poor	14 or more	10 or less	5 to 8	1 or 2

pupil to write his or her name on the protocols after the completion of the tests. The individually administered screening battery took approximately 12 to 15 minutes to finish.

Example 1

Screening Battery Summary Sheet No. 1 shows the test results for Andrew, age 5 years 11 months. Andrew was a well-developed, bright youngster who was mature for his age and who did extremely well on all three tests. But Andrew was unduly serious and seemed mildly depressed. His Bender Test protocol (Plate 37) shows rather well-drawn, neatly organized figures. His Bender Test score of 6 was good and was on the level of 7-year-old children. His excellent visual-motor perception suggested an above average mental ability.

On the VADS Test (Plate 38) Andrew obtained a Total score of 19, which was at the 85th percentile for his age level (Appendix A) and resembled the VADS Test scores of average 7-year-old children (Appendix B). The digits Andrew wrote were well formed and neatly organized. He reversed the 7 and 9, but this is common for 5½-year-old youngsters. His intersensory integration, sequencing, and recall were all outstanding.

Of particular interest was Andrew's HFD (Plate 39). It too indicated that Andrew was of above average mental ability. The drawing showed three Exceptional Items for 5½-year-olds (nostrils, pupils, two-dimensional feet). However, the HFD also revealed three Emotional Indicators (omission of mouth, no hands or fingers, short arms). These three Emotional Indicators reflect insecurity and withdrawal, and possibly passive resistance and a refusal to communicate. It is most unusual for a bright, well-functioning youngster to omit the mouth on his HFD. This sign is found most often on HFDs of children who are under considerable pressure for achievement from demanding parents. Such pressure could account for Andrew's great seriousness. The boy he drew has an expression of sadness or possible fear. A later conference with Andrew's parents confirmed the suspicion that they were setting unrealistically high standards for their son and that they were expecting more of him than he was able to achieve.

Andrew's performance on the Bender Test, the VADS Test, and the HFD all clearly showed that he was of above average mental ability and that he could be expected to be an outstanding student in the first grade. Only the HFD was able to reveal that Andrew also had emotional problems and that he was unhappy and showed signs of withdrawal and passive resistance against undue pressure from his parents. These attitudes did not manifest themselves in Andrew's behavior during the testing session since the tests were presented as "games" and did not present a pressure situation. Andrew was very responsive to encouragement and praise. His parents were urged to reduce their demands on him, and they were reassured that Andrew was highly motivated and would be an excellent student if he was given support and approval rather than pressure.

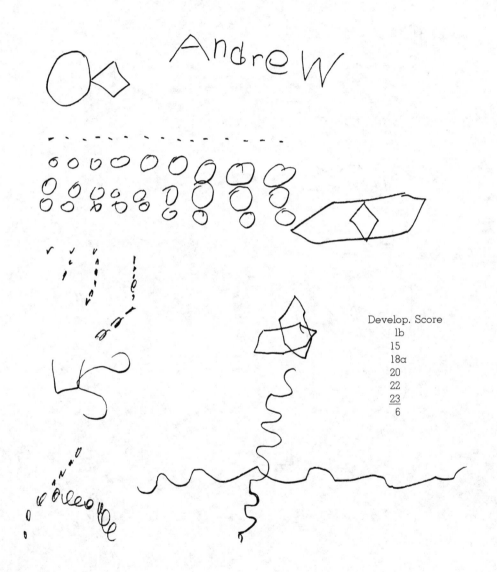

Develop. Score
lb
15
18α
20
22
23
6

Plate 37. Andrew, C.A. 5–11.

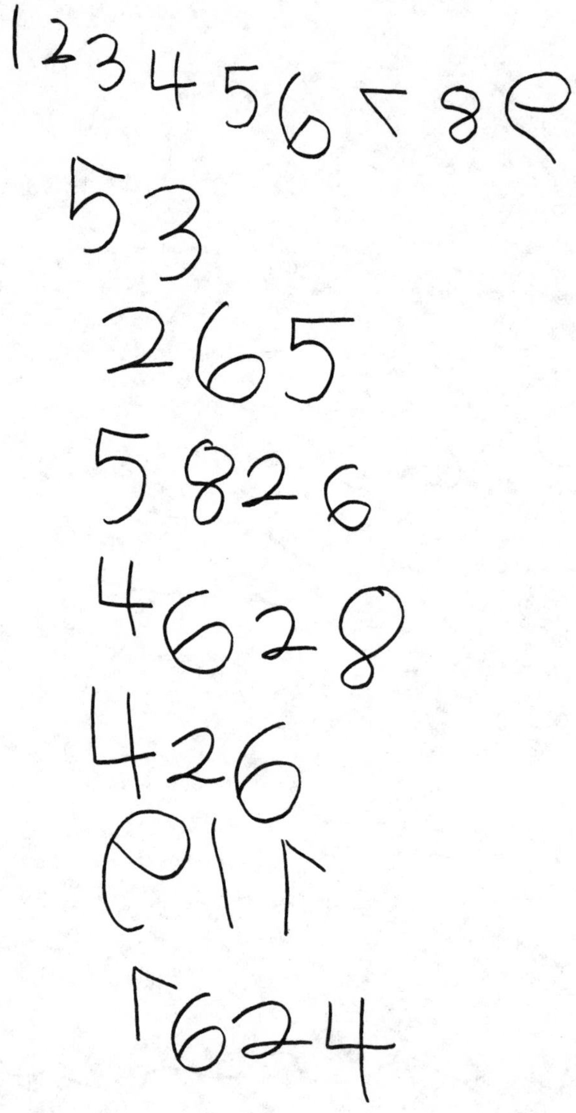

1 2 3 4 5 6 7 8 9

5 3

2 6 5

5 8 2 6

4 6 2 8

4 2 6

9 1 7

7 6 2 4

Reversals: 7, 9

Plate 38. Andrew, C.A. 5–11.

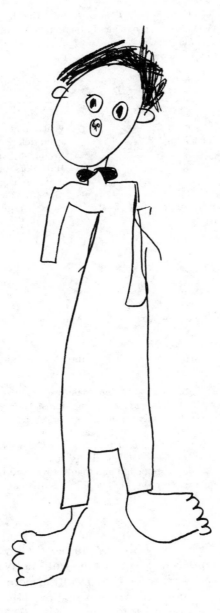

Emotional Indicators:
—omission of mouth
—no hands or fingers
—short arms

Plate 39. Andrew, C.A. 5–11.

Screening Battery Summary Sheet—Number 1

Name: Andrew   *Sex:* Male   *C.A.:* 5–11   *Time of testing:* End K (June)
Observations: Mature for age, serious, quiet, good concentration, intelligent approach to tests,
                   deliberate, careful worker
Handedness: Right   *Writing of name:* very good

Test	Score	Level	(Age equivalent)	Emotional Signs, Comments
Bender	6	High	(7–3)	good organization and control, good visual-motor perception
HFD	7	Outstanding		good details (nostrils, pupils, feet), bright, shy, insecure, 3 Emotional Indicators (omission of mouth, short arms, no hands), passive resistance to pressure?
VADS Total	19	Outstanding	(7–3)	very good intersensory integration, sequencing, and recall, good organization, well-written digits, reversal of 7 and 9, spontaneous correction of digit
Reversal	2	Average		

VADS	Score	Percentile	VADS	Score	Percentile
A–O	5	75	A I	9	83
V–O	6	75–90	V I	10	90
A–W	4	75–90	O E	11	90
V–W	4	50–75	W E	8	75
Total	19	85	Intra	9	75
			Inter	10	90

Summary: Above average mental ability, well integrated and organized, functions on 7-year
              level, however, HFD reveals emotional problems; Andrew appears to be under
              great pressure for achievement from parents or teacher; he is insecure, offers
              passive resistance, refusal to communicate, unhappy.
Recommendations: Andrew is ready for the first grade, is bright and has potential to be an
              outstanding student, but he is insecure and overly serious. It is recommended that undue
              pressure from home or school be removed and that Andrew and his parents be given
              reassurance; Andrew needs support to improve his self-esteem.

Example 2

Screening Battery Summary Sheet Number 2 shows the test results of
Kirk, age 6 years 4 months. Kirk was a tall, well-motivated youngster who
worked very slowly and with effort. He held his pencil awkwardly in his
right hand and displayed poor motor coordination. His Bender Test record
(Plate 40) showed much immaturity; it was on the level of 5-year-old children. Kirk's Bender Test score of 13 was quite low and resembled the scores
of pupils at the beginning of kindergarten. Not only were the drawings poor
but the protocol also revealed very immature organization and planning
ability. Kirk showed a tendency to perseverate (Fig. 1 and 6) and to rotate
designs (Fig. 2 and 4). Above all, he showed very poor coordination.

Poor coordination was also noted on the HFD (Plate 41), but the developmental score on the HFD was average. Kirk drew an "astronaut on the

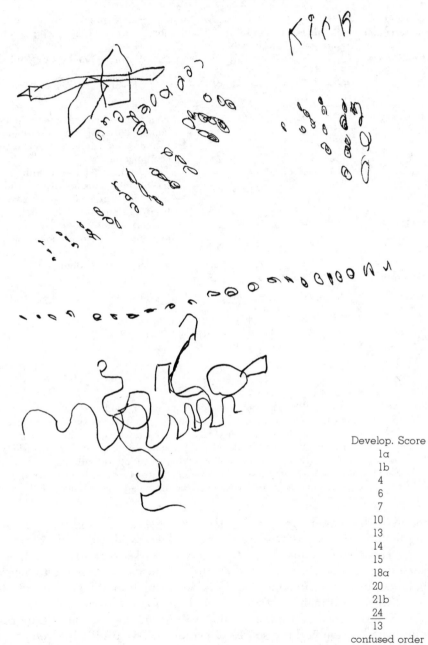

Develop. Score
1a
1b
4
6
7
10
13
14
15
18a
20
21b
24
13
confused order

Plate 40. Kirk, C.A. 6–4.

Screening Battery Summary Sheet—Number 2

Name: Kirk   *Sex:* Male   *C.A.:* 6–4   *Time of testing:* End K (June)
Observations: tall, front teeth missing, good motivation, works slowly and carefully with effort,
          holds pencil awkwardly
Handedness: Right   *Writing of name:* poor letter formation

Test	Score	Level	(Age equivalent)	Emotional Signs, Comments
Bender	13	Low	(5–1)	Poor visual-motor perception, perseveration, rotations, poor organization, poor planning, immature, poor fine-motor coordination
HFD	5	Average		"astronaut," good mental ability, anxious, poor coordination, impulsive, shading of hands and legs, could be aggressive, large hands, 2 Emotional Indicators
VADS Total	13	Average	(5–7)	difficulty writing digits, reversals, unable to write 9, poor coordination, but average visual-oral, oral expression, intrasensory integration, reads digits well.
Reversals	5	Poor	(# 2,3,5,6,7)	

VADS	Score	Percentile	VADS	Score	Percentile
A–O	4	25–50	A–I	6	25
V–O	4	50	V–I	7	38
A–W	2	10–25	O–E	8	50
V–W	3	25	W–E	5	25
Total	13	33	Intra	7	50
			Inter	6	25

Summary: Average ability, good oral expression and recall, good visual-oral integration; visual
          perception OK but immature visual-motor coordination, difficulty with writing,
          directions of digits; impulsive, disorganized, anxious, possibly aggressive.
Recommendations: Ready for first grade, average mental ability but needs help with visual-
          motor coordination, writing and direction of digits and letters, with organization and
          planning of work, and with impulse control; needs structure and support to reduce anxiety.
          Kirk's progress should be carefully watched, he may need a reassessment in the first grade.

moon"—the drawing reflected at least average mental ability. The outstanding features on the HFD were the large, heavily shaded hands and shaded legs. These signs suggest much anxiety on Kirk's part about his hands and legs; it was not certain whether this anxiety was related to aggressive behavior or to his clumsiness and poor coordination of his hands and legs.

Kirk's performance on the VADS Test (Plate 42) was uneven. His Total VADS Test score of 13 was in the average range for end-of-kindergarten pupils and resembled the scores of average 5½-year-old children (Appendix B). Once again, poor motor coordination and problems with directionality were evident. Kirk had considerable difficulty with the writing of digits. The formation of the digits was primitive, and five of them (number 2, 3, 5, 6, and 7) were reversed. Kirk was unable to write a 9. However, his Visual-Oral score was average (50th percentile), as were his Oral Expression and Intrasensory Integration scores (Appendix A). Thus, the VADS Test was able to identify Kirk's area of strength as well as his weaknesses.

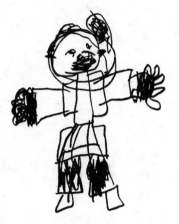

"Astronaut on the moon"

Plate 41. Kirk, C.A. 6–4.

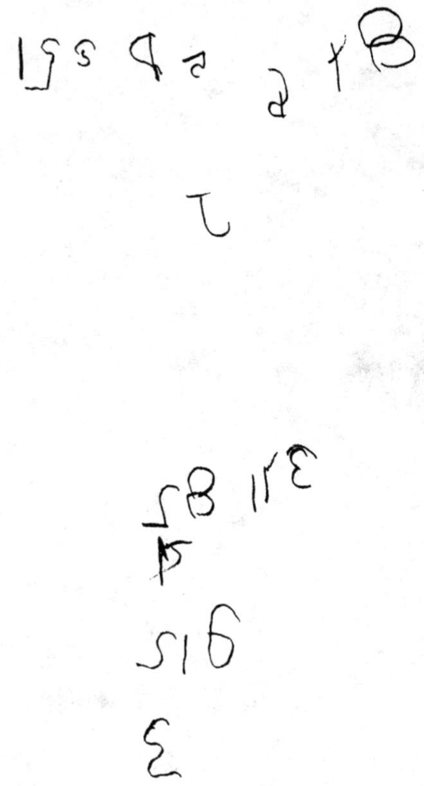

Reversals: 2, 3, 5, 6, 7
unable to write 9

Plate 42. Kirk, C.A. 6–4.

According to the HFD and VADS Test scores, Kirk was of average mental ability. All three of the screening tests showed that he had very poor motor coordination and immature visual-motor perception. But the VADS Test demonstrated that Kirk had average ability in those processes that are most closely related to school achievement, namely in visual processing, oral expression, and visual-oral integration, Kirk's performance on the screening battery suggested that he was barely ready to go to the first grade in the fall, it was recommended that he be given intensive training in visual-motor skills and help with the writing of digits and letters and with the organization of his work.

Example 3

Darryl's test scores are shown on the Screening Battery Summary Sheet Number 3. Darryl, age 6 years 1 month, was outgoing and cheerful; he worked diligently and put forth much effort to control his underlying restlessness. His speech and language were immature for his age and he had a mild articulation problem. Darryl drew the Bender Test designs with his right hand. The Bender Test record (Plate 43) revealed some constriction; Darryl placed the figures closely together in the middle portion of the paper, but the designs are well organized and the quality of the drawings are appropriate for an end-of-kindergarten pupil. Darryl's Bender Test score of 10 was average for his age and grade level. He also wrote his name quite well.

Darryl obtained a score of 5 on his HFD (Plate 44). The drawing shows good details and suggests average or possibly high average mental ability. The HFD reveals several interesting features. The large hands and the "belly button" suggest impulsivity and possible acting-out tendencies; but the large neck indicates that Darryl had learned to control his impulses. The emphasis that Darryl placed on the ears of his boy suggests that he was concerned either with things he had heard or with possible hearing difficulties on his part.

In contrast to the average Bender Test and HFD scores, Darryl's Total VADS Test score of 12 was low (Table 31). It was at the 18th percentile for 6 year olds (Appendix A) and resembled the scores of average 5-year-old-children (Appendix B). A look at Darryl's other VADS Test measures shows that his Visual-Oral and Visual Input scores were in the average range, whereas his Aural-Oral, Aural-Written, and Aural Input scores were extremely low (10th percentile). Apparently Darryl was a visual learner and had specific difficulties with auditory processing.

The digits that Darryl wrote on the VADS Test record (Plate 45) are well formed; only the 6 is reversed. But Darryl's written recall of digits was weak; he was unable to reproduce more than two digits on the Aural-Written Subtest and three digits on the Visual-Written Subtest. Darryl had no difficulty with the writing of digits, with the possible exception of the 6, but he just could not remember the digit sequences long enough to put them down on paper.

Screening Battery Summary Sheet—Number 3

Name: Darryl   *Sex:* Male   *C.A.:* 6–1   *Time of testing:* End K (June)
Observations: immature, nails severely bitten, works carefully, immature speech, mild articula-
                tion problems.
Handedness: Right   *Writing of name:* good

Test	Score	Level	(Age equivalent)	Emotional Signs, Comments
Bender	10	Average	(5–7)	Appropriate for age and grade level, good organization, perseveration, good control
HFD	5	Average		Good details (pupils, 5 fingers), average ability, good control (large neck), immature and impulsive (navel, large hands) but able to control impulsivity, emphasis on ears, possible concern about hearing or about things said
VADS Total	12	Low	(5–4)	Good written digits, good visual processing, poor aural processing, low average integration and recall
Reversals	1	High	(#6 only)	

VADS	Score	Percentile	VADS	Score	Percentile
A–O	3	10	A–I	5	10
V–O	4	50	V–I	7	38
A–W	2	10	O–E	7	25
V–W	3	25	W–E	5	25
Total	12	18	Intra	6	25
			Inter	6	25

Summary: Average mental ability, average visual-motor perception, motor coordination, orga-
            nization and control, good writing, somewhat immature intersensory integration,
            sequencing and recall, diligent worker, controlled impulsivity, poor auditory pro-
            cessing, mild articulation problem, some anxiety.
Recommendations: Ready for first grade, has average ability, visual learner, difficulty with
            auditory processing, a complete speech and hearing evaluation is recommended; Darryl's
            progress should be carefully watched, a reassessment later in the first grade is recom-
            mended.

Darryl's performance on the Bender Test and on the HFD showed that
he had average mental ability and that he was a visual learner. He did well
on the visual-motor tasks. If only the Bender Test and the HFD had been
considered, then one might have predicted that Darryl was going to be an all
around average first-grade student who would present no particular problems. However, when the results from the VADS Test were taken into
account, then the picture changed. Darryl was unquestionably a youngster of
average mental ability, but he also had areas of marked weakness. His ability
to sequence and to recall was still immature, and he showed specific problems with auditory processing. Since he also had speech and language
difficulties, and since he placed so much emphasis on the ears of the boy on
his HFD, it was recommended that he be referred for a complete speech and
hearing evaluation. It was also suggested that Darryl's progress be carefully
watched and reassessed in the first grade.

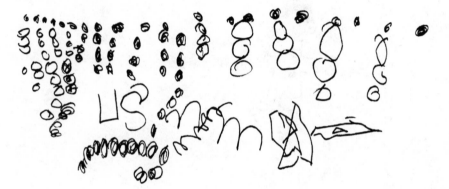

Develop. Score
1a
6
9
10
14
15
18a
21b
22
24
10

Plate 43. Darryl, C.A. 6–1.

DARRYL

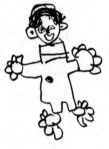

Plate 44. Darryl, C.A. 6–1.

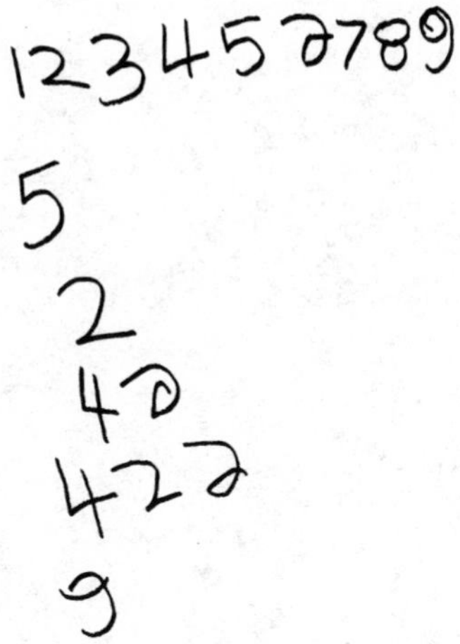

123457789

5

2

4ᴆ

42ᴆ

9

Reversal: 6

Plate 45. Darryl, C.A. 6–1.

Appendix A

Table 8.
VADS Test Percentile Scores by Age Levels

VADS	CA 5-6/5-11 (N 76) Percentile Scores					CA 6-0/6-5 (N 101) Percentile Scores				
	10	25	50	75	90	10	25	50	75	90
A-O	3	4	4	4	5	3	4	4	5	6
V-O	3	3	4	4	5	3	3	4	5	6
A-W	0	2	3	4	4	2	3	3	4	5
V-W	0	2	3	4	5	2	3	4	4	5
A I	4	6	7	8	9	5	6	4	9	10
V I	3	5	7	8	10	5	6	7	9	10
O E	6	7	8	9	10	6	7	8	10	11
W E	0	5	6	8	9	4	5	7	8	10
Intra	4	6	7	8	10	5	6	8	9	11
Inter	3	5	6	8	9	5	6	8	9	10
Total	7	11	14	16	19	10	13	15	18	20

Table 8.
VADS Test Percentile Scores by Age Levels

VADS	CA 6-6/6-11 (N 75) Percentile Scores					CA 7-0/7-11 (N 177) Percentile Scores				
	10	25	50	75	90	10	25	50	75	90
A-O	4	4	4	5	6	4	4	5	6	6
V-O	4	4	5	5	6	4	5	5	6	7
A-W	3	4	4	5	6	4	4	5	6	6
V-W	3	4	5	5	6	4	4	5	6	7
A I	7	8	8	9	11	8	8	10	11	12
V I	8	8	9	10	11	8	9	10	12	14
O E	8	8	9	10	11	8	9	10	12	13
W E	7	7	9	10	11	8	9	10	11	13
Intra	7	8	9	10	11	8	9	10	11	13
Inter	7	8	9	10	11	8	9	10	12	13
Total	15	16	18	20	22	16	18	20	23	25

Table 8. (continued)
VADS Test Percentile Scores by Age Levels

VADS	CA 8-0/8-11 (N 94) Percentile Scores					CA 9-0/9-11 (N 80) Percentile Scores				
	10	25	50	75	90	10	25	50	75	90
A-O	4	4	5	6	7	4	5	6	6	7
V-O	4	5	5	6	7	4	5	6	7	7
A-W	4	4	5	6	6	4	4	5	6	7
V-W	4	5	6	6	7	4	5	6	6	7
A I	8	9	10	11	12	8	9	11	12	13
V I	8	10	11	13	14	8	10	12	14	14
O E	9	9	11	12	13	9	10	12	13	14
W E	8	9	10	12	13	8	9	11	13	14
Intra	8	9	11	12	13	9	10	12	13	14
Inter	8	9	10	12	13	9	9	11	13	14
Total	17	19	21	23	26	17	20	23	25	27

Table 8.
VADS Test Percentile Scores by Age Levels

VADS	CA 10–0/10–11 (N 82) Percentile Scores					CA 11–0/11–11 (N 80) Percentile Scores				
	10	25	50	75	90	10	25	50	75	90
A–O	5	5	6	7	7	5	5	6	7	7
V–O	5	6	6	7	7	5	6	7	7	7
A–W	4	5	5	6	7	4	5	6	7	7
V–W	5	6	7	7	7	5	6	7	7	7
A I	9	10	12	13	13	9	11	12	13	14
V I	11	12	13	14	14	11	12	14	14	14
O E	10	11	13	13	14	10	12	13	14	14
W E	9	11	12	13	14	10	11	13	14	14
Intra	10	11	13	13	14	11	12	13	13	14
Inter	9	10	12	13	14	10	11	13	14	14
Total	20	22	25	26	27	22	23	25	27	28

Table 8. (continued)

VADS Test Percentile Scores by Age Levels

CA 12–0/12–11 (N 45)
Percentile Scores

VADS	10	25	50	75	90
A–O	5	6	6	7	7
V–O	5	6	7	7	7
A–W	5	5	6	7	7
V–W	6	7	7	7	7
A I	10	11	13	14	14
V I	12	13	14	14	14
O E	11	12	13	14	14
W E	11	12	13	14	14
Intra	11	12	13	14	14
Inter	11	12	13	14	14
Total	22	24	26	27	28

Appendix B

Total VADS Test Scores and Age Equivalents

Total VADS Score	Age Equivalents	Total VADS Scores	Age Equivalents
11	5–0 to 5–2	19	7–0 to 7–5
12	5–3 to 5–5	20	7–6 to 7–11
13	5–6 to 5–8	21	8–0 to 8–5
14	5–9 to 5–11	22	8–6 to 8–11
15	6–0 to 6–2	23	9–0 to 9–5
16	6–3 to 6–5	24	9–6 to 9–11
17	6–6 to 6–8	25	10–0 to 10–11
18	6–9 to 6–11	26	11–0 to 11–11
		27	12–0 to 12–11

Appendix C

Table 12.

VADS Test Percentile Scores by Grade Level

VADS	End of K (N 160) Percentile Scores					1st Grade (N 94) Percentile Scores				
	10	25	50	75	90	10	25	50	75	90
A–O	3	4	4	5	6	4	4	5	5	6
V–O	3	3	4	5	5	4	5	5	5	6
A–W	2	2	3	4	4	3	4	4	5	6
V–W	2	3	4	4	5	3	4	5	5	6
A I	5	6	7	8	10	7	8	9	10	12
V I	5	6	8	9	10	7	9	10	11	12
O E	6	7	8	9	11	8	9	10	11	12
W E	4	5	7	8	9	7	8	9	10	12
Intra	5	6	7	9	10	7	8	9	11	12
Inter	5	6	7	9	10	7	8	9	10	12
Total	10	12	15	17	20	15	17	18	19	23

Table 12.
VADS Test Percentile Scores by Grade Level

VADS	2nd Grade (N 121) Percentile Scores					3rd Grade (N 85) Percentile Scores				
	10	25	50	75	90	10	25	50	75	90
A–O	4	4	5	6	6	4	5	6	6	7
V–O	4	5	5	6	7	4	5	6	7	7
A–W	4	4	5	5	6	4	4	5	6	7
V–W	4	5	5	6	7	4	5	6	7	7
A I	8	9	10	11	12	8	9	10	12	13
V I	8	10	11	12	14	9	10	12	13	14
O E	9	9	11	12	13	9	10	11	12	13
W E	8	9	10	12	13	8	9	11	12	14
Intra	9	9	11	12	13	9	10	11	13	13
Inter	8	9	10	12	13	9	9	11	12	14
Total	17	19	20	23	25	18	20	22	24	27

Table 12. (continued)
VADS Test Percentile Scores by Grade Level

	4th Grade (N 69) Percentile Scores					5th Grade (N 88) Percentile Scores				
VADS	10	25	50	75	90	10	25	50	75	90
A–O	4	5	6	6	7	4	5	6	7	7
V–O	5	6	7	7	7	5	6	7	7	7
A–W	4	5	6	6	7	4	5	6	6	7
V–W	5	6	7	7	7	5	6	7	7	7
A I	9	10	11	13	14	9	10	12	13	14
V I	10	12	13	14	14	11	12	13	14	14
O E	9	11	12	13	14	10	12	13	13	14
W E	9	11	12	13	14	10	11	12	13	14
Intra	9	11	12	13	14	11	12	13	13	14
Inter	9	11	12	13	14	10	11	12	13	14
Total	19	22	24	26	27	20	22	25	26	28

Table 12.
VADS Test Percentile Scores by Grade Level

6th Grade (*N* 48)
Percentile Scores

	10	25	50	75	90
A–O	5	5	6	7	7
V–O	6	7	7	7	7
A–W	5	5	6	7	7
V–W	6	7	7	7	7
A I	9	11	12	14	14
V I	12	13	14	14	14
O E	11	12	13	14	14
W E	11	12	13	14	14
Intra	11	12	13	14	14
Inter	11	12	13	14	14
Total	22	25	25	27	28

References

Ackerman PT, Peters JE, Dykman RA: Children with specific learning disabilities: WISC profiles. J Learning Disabilities 4:33–49, 1971

Alwitt LF: Decay of immediate memory for visually presented digits among non-readers and readers. J Educ Psychol 54:144–148, 1963

Baldwin V: The relationship of Visual Aural Digit Span and Visual Aural Letter Span (VALS) to reading and spelling achievement of 20 second-grade average and 20 second-grade children with learning problems. MA thesis, University of New Mexico, 1976

Baumeister AA, Bartlett CJ: Further factorial investigations of WISC performance of Mental Defectives. Am J Ment Def 67:257–261, 1962

Baumeister AA, Bartlett CJ, Hawkins WF: Stimulus Trace as a predictor of performance. Am J Ment Def 67:726–729, 1963

Beery JW: Matching of auditory and visual stimuli by average and retarded readers. Child Development 38:827–833, 1967

Bender L: A Visual Motor Gestalt Test and its clinical use. Research Monograph No. 3. New York, American Orthopsychiatric Association, 1938

Birch HG, Belmont L: Auditory-Visual Integration in normal and retarded readers. Am J of Orthopsychiatry 34:852–861, 1964

Birch HG, Belmont L: Auditory-Visual Integration in brain-injured and normal children. Develop Med & Child Neurol 7:135–144, 1965a

Birch HG, Belmont L: Auditory-Visual Integration, intelligence and reading ability in school children. Percept Motor Skills 20:295–305, 1965b

Bridgeman B, Buttram J: Race differences on Nonverbal Analog Test performance as a function of verbal strategy training. J Educ Psychol 67(4):586–590, 1975

Carr M: Relationships between the Bender Visual Motor Gestalt Test, the Visual Aural Digit Span Test, and the Arithmetic Subtests of the Wechsler Intelligence Scale for children and the Wide Range Achievement Test. Professional paper, Texas Christian University, 1974

Carterette EC, Jones MH: Visual and auditory information processing in children and adults. Science 156:986–988, 1967

Castanada A, McCandles BR, Palermo DS: The children's form of the manifest anxiety scale. Child Development 27:317–326, 1956

Cattell RB, Scheier IH: The meaning and measurement of neuroticism and anxiety. New York: Ronald Press, 1961

Colvin AD, Koons Jr PB, Bingham JL, Fink HH: A further investigation of the relation between manifest anxiety and intelligence. J Consult Psycho 19:280–282, 1955

Comprehensive Test of Basic Skills. Monterey: CTB/McGraw Hill, 1973

Corballis MC, Loveless T: The effect of input modality on short-term serial recall. Psychon Science 7:275–276, 1967

Daehler MW, Horowitz AB, Wynns FC, Flavell JH: Verbal and nonverbal rehearsal in children's recall. Child Development 40(2):443–452, 1969

Dunn LM, Markwardt Jr FC: Peabody Individual Achievement Test Manual. Circle Pines: Am Guidance Services, 1970

Farnham-Diggory S, Gregg LW: Short-term memory function in young readers. J Exp Child Psychol 19:279–298, 1974

Finch AJ, Kendall PC, Montgomery LE: Multidimensionality of anxiety in children. J Abnorm Child Psychol 2:331–336, 1974

Finch AJ, Anderson J, Kendall PC: Anxiety and digit span performance of emotionally disturbed children. J Consult Clinical Psychol 44:874, 1976

Flanagan JC: Tests of general ability. Chicago: Science Research Associates, 1960

Flavell JH, Beach DH, Chinsky JM: Spontaneous verbal rehearsal in a memory task as a function of age. Child Development 37:283–299, 1966

Gilmore Oral Reading Test. New York: Harcourt, Brace & World, 1968

Griffiths JS: The effect of experimentally induced anxiety on certain subtests of the Wechsler-Bellevue. PhD dissertation, University of Kentucky, 1958

Guthrie JT, Goldberg HK: Visual sequential memory in reading disability. J Learning Disability 5:41–46, 1972

Hodges WF, Spielberg CD: Digit Span: An indication of trait or state anxiety? J Consult Clinical Psychol 33:430–434, 1969

Hurd AC: Visual and auditory memory testing of primary school children divided into those who are high achievers and those who are low achievers. MA thesis, San Jose State College, 1971

Jackson DN, Bloomberg R: Anxiety: Unitas or Multiplex? J Consult Psychol 22:225–227, 1958

Jastack JF, Bijou SW, Jastack SR: Wide Range Achievement Test. Wilmington: Guidance Associates, 1965

Jenkin N, Spivack G, Levine M, Savage W: Wechsler profiles and academic achievement in emotionally disturbed boys. J Consult Psychol 28:290, 1964

Johnson DS, Myklebust HR: Learning Disabilities: Educational principles and practices. New York: Grune & Stratton, 1967

Kahn D, Birch HG: Development of auditory-visual integration and reading achievement. Percept Motor Skills 27:459–468, 1968

Keeney TJ, Cannizzo SR, Flavell JH: Spontaneous and induced verbal rehearsal in a recall task. Child Development 38(4):953–966, 1967

Kirk SA, McCarthy JJ, Kirk WD: Illinois Test of Psycholinguistic Abilities. Urbana, Illinois: University of Illinois Press, 1968

Klatzky RL: Human Memory: Structures and Processes. San Francisco: WH Freeman Co, 1975

Koestler A, Jenkins JJ: Inversion effects in the tachistoscopic perception of number sequences. Psychon Sci 3:75–76, 1965

Koppitz EM: The Bender Gestalt Test for young children. New York: Grune & Stratton, 1963

Koppitz EM: Psychological evaluation of children's Human Figure Drawings. New York: Grune & Stratton, 1968

Koppitz EM: The Visual Aural Digit Span Test with elementary school children. J Clin Psychol 26:349–353, 1970

Koppitz EM: Children with learning disabilities: A five year follow-up study. New York: Grune & Stratton, 1971

Koppitz EM: The Visual Aural Digit Span Test performance of boys with emotional and learning problems. J Clin Psychol 29:463–466, 1973

Koppitz EM: The Bender Gestalt Test for young children. Volume II, Research and application, 1963–1973. New York: Grune & Stratton, 1975a

Koppitz EM: Bender Gestalt Test, Visual Aural Digit Span Test and reading achievement. J Learning Disability 8:154–157, 1975b

Koppitz EM: Visual Aural Digit Span Test Stimulus Cards. New York: Grune & Stratton, 1977a

Koppitz EM: Visual Aural Digit Span Test Scoring Sheet. New York: Grune & Stratton, 1977b

Leslie L: Susceptibility to interference effects in short-term memory of normal and retarded readers. Percept Motor Skills 40(3):791–794, 1975

Lindner R, Fillmer H: Auditory and visual performance of slow readers. The Reading Teacher 24:16–22, 1970

London P, Robinson JP: Imagination in learning and retention. Child Development 39:803–815, 1968

Lyle JG, Goyen J: Visual recognition, developmental lag, and strephosymbolia in reading retardation. J Abnorm Psychol 73:25–29, 1968

Mahoney TP: Visual short-term memory in retarded and normal children. PhD dissertation, Rutgers State University, 1972

Matarazzo RG: The relationship of manifest anxiety to Wechsler-Bellevue Subtest performance. J Consult Psychol 19:218, 1955

Meeker MN: Immediate memory and its correlates with school achievement. PhD dissertation, University of Southern California, 1966

Millavec MM: The performance of negro and caucasian children on specific linguistic and sequential tasks. MA Thesis, San Jose State College, 1971

Miller GA: The magical number seven, plus or minus two: Some limits on our capacity for processing information. Psychol Review 63:81–97, 1956

Moldowsky S, Moldowsky PC: Digit span as anxiety indicator. J Consult Psychol 16:115–118, 1952

Morea WJ: private communication, Commack, New York, 1976

Murray DJ, Roberts B: Visual and auditory presentation, presentation rate and short-term memory in children. Brit J Psychol 59:119–125, 1968

Nalven FB: Relationship between digit span and distractibility ratings in emotionally disturbed children. J Clin Psychol 23:466–467, 1967

Pyke S, Agnew NMcK: Digit Span performance as a function of noxious stimulation. J. Consult Psychol 27:28, 1963

Rose FC: The occurrence of short auditory memory span among school children referred for diagnosis of reading difficulties. J Educ Research 51:459–464, 1958

Rubin B: Cupertino, California: private communication, 1974

Rudel RG, Teuber HL: Pattern recognition within and across sensory modalities in normal and brain injured children. Neuropsychologia 9:389–399, 1971

Rudisill M: Flashed digit and phrase recognition of oral and concrete responses: A study of advanced and retarded readers in the third grade. J Psychol 42:317–328, 1956

Samuels SJ, Anderson RH: Visual recognition memory, paired associate learning, and reading achievement. J Educ Psychol 65(2):160–167, 1973

Senf GM: Development of immediate memory for bisensory stimuli in normal children and children with learning disorders. Develop Psychol Monograph 1(6), Part 2, 1969

Shumar LS: The relationship of the Visual Aural Digit Span Test to reading achievement for lower elementary school children. MA Thesis, University of Akron, 1976

Siegel S: Nonparametric statistics. New York: McGraw-Hill Book Co., 1956

Silberberg NE, Silberberg MC: Hyperlexia: Special word recognition skills in young children. Exceptional Children 34:41–42, 1967

Simon HA: How big is a chunk? Science 183:483–488, 1974

Sperling G: The information available in brief visual presentation. Psychol Monograph 74(11), whole No 498, 1960

Spielberger CD: Theory and research on anxiety. In Spielberger CD (Ed): Anxiety and behavior. New York: Academic Press, 1966

Spitz HH: A note on immediate memory for digits: Invariance over the years. Psychol Bulletin 78: 183–185, 1972

Spitz HH, LaFontaine L: The Digit Span of Idiot Savants. Am J Ment Defic 77: 757–759, 1973

Spring C: Encoding speed and memory span in dyslexic children. J Spec Educ 10:35–40, 1976

Taylor JA: A personality scale of manifest anxiety. J Abnorm Soc Psychol 48:285–290, 1953

Terman LM, Merrill M: Stanford-Binet Intelligence Scales. Boston: Houghton-Mifflin, 1960

Thompson GC: The relationship between the VADS Test and selected measures of reading. MA thesis, University of Akron, 1976

Tiegs EW, Clark WW: California Achievement Tests Examiners' Manual. Monterey: CTB/ McGraw-Hill, 1970

Tulving E: Subjective organization and effects of repetition on multi-trial free-recall learning. J Verbal Learn & Verbal Behav 5:193–197, 1966

Wachs T. Free-recall learning in children as a function of chronological age, intelligence and motivational orientation. Child Development 40(2):577–589, 1969

Wakefield WM: Sequential memory responses in normal and clinical readers. Elementary English 50:939–940, 1973

Wechsler D: Wechsler Intelligence Scale for Children. New York: The Psychological Corporation, 1949

Wechsler D: The measurement and appraisal of adult intelligence. Baltimore: The Williams & Wilkins Co., 1958

Wechsler D: Wechsler Intelligence Scale for Children—Revised. New York: The Psychological Corporation, 1974

Witkin BR: Reading improvement through auditory perceptual training. Alameda County Schools, Hayward, California, 1971

Index